"This fine book elucidates the characteristics of communication in a Japanese residential care institution through the author's analysis of linguistic interaction between carers and residents during the morning care segment of their day. Its timely and thoughtful approach to the multifaceted linguistic issues involved in caring for residents in a rapidly expanding sector which is also dealing with the introduction of foreign care workers and moves towards robotic care assistants makes a very valuable contribution to the growing literature in this field."

– **Emeritus Professor Nanette Gottlieb**,
School of Languages and Cultures, The University of Queensland

"Care Communication is a challenge to all eldercare institutions to take moment-by-moment verbal interactions between staff and residents seriously, if they are to claim care for their residents' well-being. As Backhaus notes in his closing chapter '. . . the overall importance of communication to institutional eldercare is by no means as obvious to care professionals as it may be to the linguist or social scientist'. But after reading this book, it will be. Care Communication is a methodologically sound, theoretically informed, and clearly written account – from multiple possible angles of analytic perspectives – of the verbal techniques of control and resistance that perfuse the daily talk between caregivers and care recipients at a single Japanese eldercare facility. Its conclusions are compelling and the implications for our understanding of how well-being is (or is not) built in daily micro-encounters between staff and residents make this an indispensable addition to the study of eldercare institutions in particular and of institutional communication in general."

– **Professor Emerita Janet S. Shibamoto-Smith**,
Department of Anthropology, University of California, Davis

Care Communication

This book studies communication in institutional eldercare. It is based on audio-recorded interactions between residents and staff in a Japanese care facility. The focus is on the morning care routines, which include getting the residents out of bed and ready for the day. Combining quantitative and qualitative methods, the analysis explores the characteristics of care communication as they become manifest in the interactional small print. Topics include the use of terms of address and formal speech, the basic organisation of openings and closings, the difficulties of talking while working – and, at times, working while talking – and tempo differences between residents and staff as they move along between bed and breakfast. The research findings are contextualised with results from previous studies, tracing significant features and explanation for deviant cases.

The author is a trained linguist and certified nursing assistant with first-hand working experience in institutional eldercare.

Peter Backhaus is Professor at Waseda University, Tokyo. His main research interests are sociolinguistics, pragmatics, and writing and orthography. Publications include *Linguistic Landscapes: A Comparative Study of Urban Multilingualism in Tokyo* (Multilingual Matters, 2007) and *Communication in Elderly Care: Cross-cultural Perspectives* (ed., Continuum, 2011).

Routledge Studies in Sociolinguistics

For a full list of titles in this series, please visit www.routledge.com

Care Communication

Making a Home in a Japanese
Eldercare Facility

Peter Backhaus

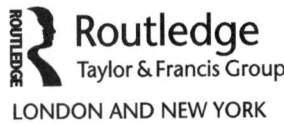 Routledge
Taylor & Francis Group

LONDON AND NEW YORK

First published 2017 by Routledge
2 Park Square, Milton Park, Abingdon, Oxon OX14 4RN

605 Third Avenue, New York, NY 10017

First issued in paperback 2021

Routledge is an imprint of the Taylor & Francis Group, an informa business

Publisher's Note
The publisher has gone to great lengths to ensure the quality of
this reprint but points out that some imperfections in the
original copies may be apparent.

British Library Cataloguing-in-Publication Data
A catalogue record for this book is available from the British Library

Library of Congress Cataloging-in-Publication Data
Names: Backhaus, Peter, 1975– author.
Title: Care communication : making a home in a Japanese
    eldercare facility / by Peter Backhaus.
Description: Abingdon, Oxon ; New York, NY : Routledge, 2017. |
    Series: Routledge studies in sociolinguistics ; 14 | Includes
    bibliographical references and index.
Identifiers: LCCN 2016049081 | ISBN 9781138229846 (hardback) |
    ISBN 9781315387826 (ebook)
Subjects: LCSH: Older people—Care—Japan. | Older people—
    Communication—Japan. | Communication in nursing—Japan. |
    Nursing homes—Japan.
Classification: LCC HV1484.J32 B33 2017 | DDC 362.610952—dc23
LC record available at https://lccn.loc.gov/2016049081

ISBN 13: 978-0-367-41066-7 (pbk)
ISBN 13: 978-1-138-22984-6 (hbk)

Typeset in Galliard
by Apex CoVantage, LLC

Contents

Figures

Tables

Foreword

In the conclusion to our handbook chapter on discourse and aging, Toshiko Hamaguchi and I argue that in order to make sense of the intricate relationship between discourse and aging and sufficiently appreciate the heterogeneity of the elderly population, we need to 'continue to *carry out studies of well-defined subgroups of the aging population who are engaged in specific activities in specific settings*'. Following Coupland (2009: 851), we hold that aging needs to be treated 'as something we achieve in the minutiae of our social lives, in social encounters of diverse sorts and even in individual acts of expression in speech and writing'. With reference to Becker's (1984) notion of particularity, we stress that it is only through attention to detail that we will arrive at more general insights, since 'each of these two areas – aging and discourse – is so large and multifaceted as to preclude any real understanding of their interconnections if each is not broken down into manageable parts' (Hamilton and Hamaguchi 2015: 719).

As if in response to our plaidoyer, Peter Backhaus has written a beautifully illustrated characterization of the power of language within the minutiae that together construct the interactions involving 25 residents and 6 care workers that occur within a geriatric health care facility in the outskirts of Tokyo, Japan. In order to discern meaning within this highly complex environment, he focuses our attention on 107 audio-recorded morning care interactions during what is 'arguably the busiest time of day' in the facility, as the participants 'work their way from bed to breakfast'.

In the process, Backhaus conducts both delicate qualitative and fine-grained quantitative analyses from the frameworks of conversation analysis and interactional sociolinguistics to illuminate the use of honorifics (chapter 4); the coordination of openings and closings of these social encounters (chapter 5); the complicated relationship between 'task work' and 'talk work', as activities related to 'bed and body work' (Gubrium 1975: 125) are performed (chapter 6); and the differences between the 'operation speed' of the care workers and the preferred tempo of the residents (chapter 7). All this work leads in a sophisticated way to our enhanced understanding of three basic attributes of eldercare communication as displayed in the morning care procedures of the care facility: (1) focused on the tasks; (2) asymmetrical; and (3) performed in a constant hurry.

The pages of Backhaus' book are filled with analytical gems far too numerous to mention here; his insights are connected to an astonishing number of relevant published studies and offer us poignant glimpses into a world most of us will never know with this level of particularity. I personally was most taken with Backhaus' exquisite examination of the ways in which tempo differences between residents and staff manifest themselves 'in the small print of the interactional give and take', producing a pervasive hurriedness throughout the morning care activities. This is but one of myriad findings in this book that are both intriguing to scholars and relevant to professional practice.

The final subheading of the book's concluding chapter reads 'Who cares?' I laughed aloud when I came upon it, fully recognizing my own voicing of this question in many of my cross-disciplinary research projects and consultations with health care practitioners. How very challenging it can be to make transparent the critical nature of language in discussions with those trained to view problems through very different lenses. But as I turned the final page and my spirits soared with a sense that I had learned so very much through my engagement with this book, I can confidently answer that ubiquitous question: *I* do. I *do* care. And undoubtedly readers of this fine study will echo my response.

Heidi E. Hamilton

Acknowledgements

'If this had been your PhD thesis, it would have ruined your career', said a colleague of mine, in view of the rather large amount of time it took to get this book ready. I tend to see it just the other way round – that my 'career' almost ruined the book – but I know this is a poor excuse for delayed delivery. That I finally did deliver is due to a great number of people, whose friendliness, cooperation, advice, support, encouragement, and endurance I gratefully acknowledge.

First of all, I have to thank everyone at Edogawa Care, especially the residents and staff on the second floor, who allowed me to observe and record their manifold interactions during the morning care activities. I'm infinitely grateful to them for allowing me a glimpse into their everyday lives and their various ways of caring for each other.

Florian Coulmas has been supportive of this project from its very start, in many functions including superior, supervisor, and friend. Heidi E. Hamilton provided much personal and professional encouragement, and a foreword that is definitely the best thing that could happen to this book. Ayako Shikama supported me during the data collection and substantially helped with the transcripts. Particularly during these early parts of the project, it was very 'healthy' to have someone to talk to who was just as into the data as I was.

Various fully, semi-, and non-anonymous reviewers took the time to read parts of the text and provide critical feedback, including Florian Coulmas and Hiroaki Izumi, both of whom worked through the whole manuscript, Tomoko Furuta, Keiko Kitamoto, Heidi E. Hamilton, Boyd Davis, and John C. Maher, who also helped with the title.

Other colleagues whose diverse ways of support I would like to acknowledge, hopefully not missing out too many, are Charles Antaki, Laurence Anthony, Yong-Ik Bak, Andrew Barke, Oana David, Julian Dierkes, Agnes M. Engbersen, Eileen Fairhurst, Sigrid Francke, Sage Lambert Graham, Masato Harikae, Claus Harmer, Trine Heinemann, Barbara Holthus, Carola Hommerich, Hiromichi Hosoma, Ian Hutchby, Andrew James, Gunilla Jansson, Florian Kohlbacher, Anna Lindström, Gabriele Lucius-Hoene, Yoshiko Matsumoto, Kumiko Murata, Kunihiko Muto, Yukako Nozawa, Sae Oshima, Takao Onoda, André Posenau, Karen Shire, Yuko Sugita, Rie Suzuki, Kimie Ueno, and my friend Fritz, for making it all possible.

I gratefully acknowledge support by the German Institute for Japanese Studies (www.dijtokyo.org), where I was based during the earlier stages of this project, and by Waseda University (www.waseda.jp), where I am now.

Thanks as always to my family, who had to make do with some substantial lack of 'care' while I was working on this book. I apologise.

Tokyo, September 2016

1 Introduction

I first got 'admitted' to an eldercare institution at a comparatively young age. I was 18 at the time, and had just finished high school in a small town in what was formerly known as West Germany. It was 1994 and the Cold War officially over, but my newly reunited country was still anxious to keep its conscription system going. Luckily for those who felt little inclination to serve in the army, there was a so-called 'civilian service' that included various types of community work. Thus I was able to trade in my one year of military service for 15 months of employment as a care assistant in an old people's home.

Whereas many of my 'draft dodging' friends had got themselves relatively easy-going jobs as meals on wheels drivers, caretakers, or municipal office assistants, I all of a sudden found myself among wheelchairs and hospital beds, toilets and bedpans, clean and dirty linen, and many people two or three generations my senior. Getting along in these new circumstances was quite a challenge, both physically and emotionally, not least for a fresh high school graduate with no previous work experience whatsoever. And though I kept telling myself throughout these 15 months that it was all a most valuable experience – which it certainly was! – I was glad when I had finally done my time and was 'discharged' into normal adult life.

The project described in this book brought me back into eldercare more than a decade later. In autumn 2005, I had just finished my PhD and started a job at a German research institute in Tokyo, which by the time was conducting a larger interdisciplinary project on Japan's recent demographic developments. I was entrusted with doing 'the linguistic part' of it, whatever that was supposed to be. Faced with a most welcome freedom of topic choice, I quickly decided I should get back to my previous civilian service experiences, and so started my second, slightly less applied approach to institutional eldercare.

As I will describe in chapter 3, it turned out somewhat more difficult this time to find an institution that would allow me in. However, once I had been granted access, I found that many of the things I saw felt strangely familiar. Despite being a cultural outsider with little to no first-hand knowledge of Japanese healthcare settings, I realised that the people involved, both residents and staff, were faced with very similar issues as I had experienced them during my one-time care worker career in Germany: how to cope with growing dependence and loss of autonomy; how to reconcile individual preferences with institutional rules and regulations; how to keep a healthy adult distance while having to engage in most intimate activities with each other; how to navigate between institutional and personal identities; and, generally speaking, how to make a home in a place that is so much unlike home. A large part of these issues are worked out through language. This is, in a nutshell, what this book is about.

In what follows, I will examine the nature of care communication from a sociolinguistic perspective. The next chapter starts with an overview of the socio-political background to eldercare in Japan and the dramatic demographic developments creating this background. It gives the most recent figures on the quickly growing number of people in need of care and the types of services they use. The second section introduces the main characteristics of care communication as they have been identified in previous studies. This is accompanied by an up-to-date review of the small but growing body of research on the topic in Japanese. The chapter closes with a few comparative observations about similarities and differences between research in Japan and research in other cultural contexts.

In chapter 3, I describe how the data for the present study were collected and compiled into a sample of 107 morning care interactions. These form the corpus on which the analysis in the subsequent chapters is based. The research question that will guide us through this study is: What are the main characteristics of resident–staff interaction during the morning care activities in the setting under observation? I preview the methods and analytical tools applied to answer this question, closing with a few critical remarks on methodological issues.

Chapter 4 is the first in a series of four main chapters dedicated to the analysis of the data. Dealing with honorifics, it starts with a few opening remarks on the topic and the connection (and growing disconnect) between honorifics and politeness. The first section zooms in on terms of address. It identifies predominant patterns in address term usage by the participants, but also discusses some deviant cases and what they interactionally achieve. Section 2 looks at speech level as the most prominent type of Japanese addressee honorifics. The quantitative analysis shows that both residents and care workers mostly use a non-formal speech style, though it also reveals that there are greater individual differences. A closer inspection of single cases further illustrates the important discourse-organising function of shifts between plain and formal speech, which is largely in line with more recent research on the topic. Section 3 explores various types of referent honorifics, including archaic forms like *gozaru* and how they are used for the sake of humour and verbal play.

The analysis in chapter 5 is divided into two parts that examine the opening and closing of morning care interaction, respectively. As to the former, a set of constitutive elements is identified that are commonly part of an opening, including a preparation phase, a summons, a greeting, and some reference to the reason for a care worker's attending to a resident. Various excerpts are presented to show how the participants need to work through these components to prepare the ground for the beginning of the physical tasks. The second half of the chapter explores how a care worker and resident manage to 'un-meet' by bringing an interaction to an orderly end. The analysis shows that the prototypical components of closing sequences as identified in previous research are recognisable in the present data, too. However, the task-oriented nature of the interactions requires them to be addressed in substantially different ways. While both the openings and the closings are characterised by the care workers' control of the interactional flow, the chapter also presents two deviating cases that show how a reversal of the turn structure can substantially increase a resident's degree of agency.

Chapter 6 is the longest and, in many respects, central chapter of the analysis. Based on previous research, it starts with a distinction between task talk and non-task talk. Task-talk is defined as talk that directly relates to a care task, whereas non-task talk has no immediate relevance to the running tasks. A detailed analysis of task talk is provided in the first section, which deals with control acts, inquiry sequences, transition markers, and heave-hoes. The second part of the chapter explores non-task talk, the most frequent topics residents and staff talk about, and the differing topic preferences of the two groups. Based on the first two sections, the third part examines shifts between task talk and non-task talk and the interactional difficulties that come with such shifts. A closer analysis of single cases also shows how shifts to non-task talk can entail a re-definition of the participants' roles beyond the institutional frame.

In chapter 7, I demonstrate how different tempo preferences of the care workers and the residents become manifest in the interactional flow of the exchanges. Three interrelated phenomena are discussed, each of which is analysed in a separate section. Section 1 explores overlaps that result from 'delayed' delivery of a resident's pending utterance. Section 2 focuses on the care workers' common practice of repeating words or phrases within a single turn. A closer inspection of these so-called 'multiple sayings' shows that they may be used to either speed up a required action by a resident or prevent moves considered premature. The third section deals with the repetition of full turns, regularly used by the care workers to call for delivery of a resident's 'missing' verbal reaction. From a quantitative perspective, one surprising point is that in many cases, the verbal reaction is in fact delivered without any delay, but for some reason goes unnoticed by the busy care worker. This suggests that a high interactional tempo may in fact result in a slower performance of the tasks.

The concluding chapter reviews the main findings of the study. Returning to the research question, it identifies three main characteristics of care communication, derived from the data analysis and largely in line with findings from previous studies in different cultural contexts. These are (1) task-orientedness, (2) interactional asymmetry, and (3) time pressure. After reviewing each point in detail, the findings are discussed in the light of two larger sociolinguistic issues: gender and im/politeness. The book concludes with a few personal reflections on the role of communication in eldercare. A detailed table of contents is provided in Appendix 2.

The data analysis contains a total of 46 transcripts from the recorded data, which are in the centre of the analysis in the main chapters. All transcripts are largely based on Jefferson's transcription system (Atkinson and Heritage 1984: ix–xvi, Jefferson 2004), which provides a standardised set of rules for producing written representations of spoken interaction. A complete list of the symbols and abbreviations used in the transcripts is given in Appendix 1.

Romanisation of all Japanese terms is based on the modified Hepburn system (SWET 1998). Long vowels are marked with macrons, except for material quoted from the transcripts, where, following common practice, the vowel is doubled. Insertion of space between words is motivated by reasons of readability. Select morphemes such as *san* (person suffix) or *o* (beautification prefix) are attached using hyphens. All translations have been done by myself.

2 Background and previous research

This chapter sets out to provide the larger background to care communication. We start with a brief outline of Japan's recent demographic developments and how they relate to an increasing interest in the topic of eldercare in general, and the role of communication in particular. This is followed by a review of previous research, divided into two parts. Section 2.2 introduces the sociolinguistic background and summarises the main findings from research on communication in eldercare outside Japan, while section 2.3 takes a closer look at the available literature on research in Japanese settings. Rather than focusing on cultural specifics, it will be shown that previous studies across the globe have come across a couple of noteworthy similarities – to which we will come back more than once during the analysis in the later chapters.

2.1 Eldercare in Japan

Japanese demographics regularly hit the news. With a median age of 46.1 years and an average life expectancy of over 83 years, present-day Japan can pride itself with what is most likely the oldest population a country in the world has ever had. And it got there with remarkable speed: Whereas back in 1970, people 65 or older made up a mere 7% of the total population, their share is up to 27.5% today, and counting. According to predictions by the National Institute of Population and Social Security Research, it will reach almost 40% by 2060 (IPSS 2016: Table 2–8). This 'demographic time bomb', as some call it (e.g., Goto 2014), poses great challenges to the social and economic conditions under which the country operates (Coulmas et al. 2008), including its welfare and social security systems (Thang 2011). Needless to say, providing care for an ever growing share of the population is one of the major issues.

As in many societies, older people in Japan traditionally were looked after by their families. It was expected that the eldest son after marriage would move in with his parents and take care of them in their later years. In effect, this put the main burden on the daughter-in-law, who bore the chief responsibility for the care of older household members (Sodei 1995, Jenike 2003). However, a trend towards nuclear families and an increase of single-person households has gradually turned such arrangements obsolete. Although co-residence with one's older parents or in-laws is still more common in Japan than in most western societies (Linhart 1997, Orpett Long and Harris 1997), home-based care is becoming increasingly hard to provide.

It took Japanese society and its law-making representatives some time to let go of the idea of family-based care and overcome the social stigma attached to care institutions in general. One major impediment to change was that institutionalisation for a long time was associated with the legend of *ubasuteyama*, a mountain where older household members were abandoned to die when becoming a burden to the community at large (Bethel 1992a: 112, 1992b: 130–131, Wu 2004: 11).

Such negative images notwithstanding, a series of laws since the 1980s have worked towards a substantial reorganisation of the welfare system and an overall "socialisation of care" (Coulmas 2007: chapter 6, also see Campbell 2000, Peng 2008). Most far-reaching among these changes was the introduction of the Long Term Care Insurance System (*kaigo hoken seido*, LTC) in 2000, which, according to Orpett Long (2008: 201), 'voiced a radical departure from previous cultural assumptions about family care giving'.

The LTC system is a mandatory, premium-based insurance scheme that provides a wider range of home help and institutional nursing and day care services (see, e.g., Ozawa and Nakayama 2005, IPSS 2014: 33–41). It has been intended to de-hospitalise care, which by the end of the 1980s had become a serious social and financial problem, and 'encourage older people to live with a minimum of dislocation and a maximum of independence as long as possible' (Kingston 2011: 74). The system is geared towards the development and use of community-based services (Morikawa 2014), a move Shimada and Tagsold (2006: 159) assess as a 'somewhat mechanical' type of solidarity. Although the LTC system faces major challenges, financial and other, public opinion overall has been favourable (Yong and Saito 2012).

The latest figures available from the Japanese Ministry of Health, Labour and Welfare (MHLW 2016a) show that as of 2014, over 5 million people were using services covered by the LTC system. As can be seen in Figure 2.1, the majority were receiving some sort of at-home service, with regular visits by home helpers or other medical professionals, or were frequenting day care centres, which provide meals, physical exercise, and recreational activities. Around 18%, or a total of 900,000 people, were living in one of various types of care facilities, showing that residential care is becoming a reality for a growing number of Japan's older population.

The high popularity of the LTC system has entailed a severe shortage of residential care facilities. Particularly the urban population is faced with long waiting lists and a large number of so-called *kaigo nanmin*, care vagabonds (literally, 'care refugees') desperately looking for admission into long-time institutional care. A related problem is the chronic shortage of qualified care workers. Harsh working conditions and low pay have kept the numbers of new applicants in this occupational sector low, and turnover rates rampant (Ohwa and Chen 2012, Aoki 2016). As Japanese sociologist Chizuko Ueno (2011)

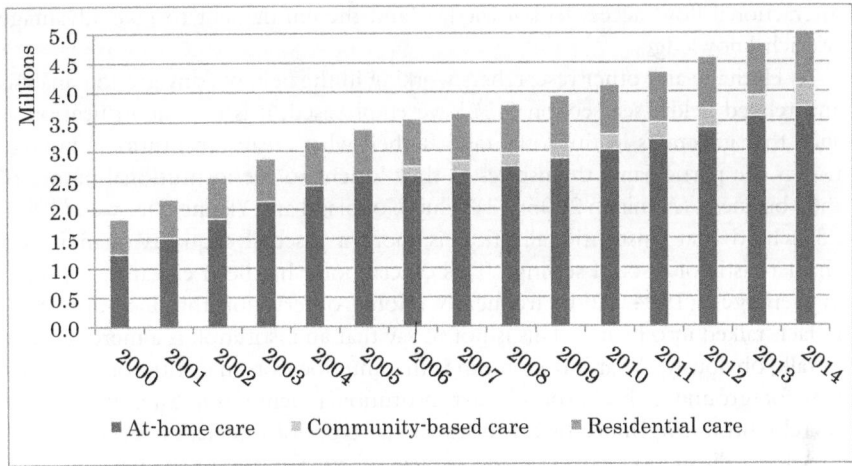

Figure 2.1 Total number and type of service used by LTC care recipients, 2000–2014 (MHLW 2016a). No later data available as of August 2016.

has pointed out, care work in Japan is still lacking appropriate social and financial recognition.

Recently discussed strategies to deal with the problem of labour shortage in the care sector include the promotion of robot technologies (e.g., Nagakura 2016), the assignment of elderly residents from the capital region to care facilities in outlying prefectures (Masuda 2015), and the admission of foreign care workers to the domestic job market, for which bilateral economic partnership agreements (EPAs) were concluded with Indonesia, the Philippines, and Vietnam (Vogt 2009, Akashi 2014). As will be shown in section 2.3, these developments have left their mark on recent research into communication in Japanese eldercare (e.g., Takamoto 2011). Before taking a closer look at the Japanese literature though, it is necessary to sketch out the overall sociolinguistic background and briefly outline the main findings from research on care communication in general.

2.2 Care and communication

The topic of communication in eldercare cuts into two comparatively well-researched subfields in sociolinguistics and discourse studies: institutional interaction and communication with older adults. Starting with the former, Heritage (e.g., 1997, 2004) has summarised a number of aspects through which the 'institutionality' of institutional interaction becomes manifest. These include common patterns of turn-taking and turn design, a structural organisation that in many cases falls into identifiable 'goal- and task-oriented sections', lexical choices that come with the reiterative nature of institutional encounters, and asymmetries between the participants with respect to the right to determine the interactional flow, access to knowledge, and the entitlement to take advantage of such knowledge.

As Heritage and other researchers working in the field of conversation analysis and related fields (see section 3.3) have emphasised, it is not the institution as such that generates institutional talk. Rather, what creates institutional interaction is the participants themselves as they 'orient to the institutional nature of their business' (Arminen 2005: 32). Thus Coupland and Ylänne-McEwen (1993: 233) hold that 'institutionalization is more a discursive quality than it is a characteristic of a social setting'. This crucial point has been elegantly captured in Heritage's (1984a: 290) frequently quoted observation that institutions are in fact 'talked into being'. This is not to say that an institution is a mere product of talk, obviously. What it does mean is that interlocutors in institutional settings may foreground or background their institutional identities in a variety of ways, thereby producing more or less institutional types of interaction as they talk.

A basic distinction can be made between formal and informal types of institutional settings (Drew and Heritage 1992: 25–29). The former include classrooms, courtrooms, and news interviews. All of these tend to follow a strictly regulated system of turn-taking, deviation from which may be subject to sanctioning. Non-formal settings allow for a freer and more variegated distribution of turns that may in many instances 'approximate conversational or at least "quasi-conversational" modes' (Drew and Heritage 1992: 28). This applies to workplace settings, service encounters, and most medical contexts, including eldercare institutions like the one examined in this study.

Notwithstanding the 'loose' nature of their micro-level structure, care facilities are commonly classified as a type of 'total institution'. According to Goffman (1961: xiii), this is 'a place of residence and work where a large number of like-situated individuals, cut off from the wider society for an appreciable period of time, together lead an enclosed, formally administered round of life'. Apart from several sorts of care facilities, Goffman (1961: 4–12) distinguishes a number of other types of total institutions, including mental hospitals, prisons, army barracks, and monasteries. Common to them is a breakdown of the social and physical separations among 'sleep, play, and work', the bureaucratic organisation of everyday life, systematic surveillance of the 'inmates', and incompatibility of the institution with any form of family life. Though Goffman's own research never specifically zoomed in on eldercare, his concept of the total institution has served as a point of reference to many subsequent researchers studying interaction in this setting (e.g., Gubrium 1975, Gibb 1990, Coupland and Ylänne-McEwen 1993, Grainger 1993a, 1993b, Hamilton 1994, Somera 1995, Salari and Rich 2001, Makoni and Grainger 2002, Wu 2004, Salari 2005, Williams and Warren 2009, Marson and Powell 2014).

This brings us to the second relevant topic, communication with older adults. The process of ageing entails a variety of changes in an individual's linguistic competence that need to be taken into account (Thornton and Light 2006, Burke and Shafto 2008, Wright 2016). Apart from real cognitive deficits, however, research in sociolinguistics and social psychology has emphasised that attitudes about these deficits may exercise a major influence on how communication between younger and older adults, both impaired and healthy, is shaped.

Studies on intergenerational communication in institutional and non-institutional settings have identified specific ways of speaking called 'patronising talk' or 'elderspeak'. According to Hummert and Ryan (1996), patronising talk is motivated by the dialectic between caring and controlling attitudes, and consists of four interrelated elements: (1) directive talk (e.g., use of directives, swearing, shouting), (2) baby talk (e.g., use of diminutives and endearments, see also Caporael 1981, Caporael et al. 1983, Ryan et al. 1994, O'Connor and Rigby 1996), (3) overly personal talk (e.g., excessive praise), and (4) superficial talk (e.g., through particular topic choices). As Coupland and Ylänne-McEwen (2006: 2336) acknowledge, patronising talk 'may stem from very positive relational goals such as showing care, concern and nurturance'. However, due to the inherent component of control, patronising talk has also been discussed in relation to the topic of impoliteness (e.g., Hummert and Mazloff 2001). We will come back to this problem in chapter 8.

Since the 1980s, a small but growing number of empirical studies have explored naturally occurring interaction between care recipients and care professionals in various cultural contexts. Focusing on studies available in English, there is now research from the US (Smithers 1977, Caporael 1981, Kayser-Jones 1981, Wagnild and Manning 1985, Nussbaum 1993, Dijkstra et al. 2002, Carpiac-Claver and Levy-Storms 2007, McLean 2007, Davis et al. 2016) and Canada (Jones and Jones 1986), the UK (Lipman et al. 1979, Wells 1980, Fairhurst 1981, Kayser-Jones 1981, Grainger 1990, 1993a, 1993b, 1998, 2004a, Grainger et al. 1990, Thomas 1992, Hewison 1995, Ward et al. 2008), Australia (Gibb 1990, Gibb and O'Brien 1990, Edwards et al. 2003) and New Zealand (Maclagan and Grant 2011, Marsden and Holmes 2014), as well as from Sweden (Hallberg et al. 1993, Skovdahl et al. 2003, Lindström 2005, Wadensten 2005, Jansson and Plejert 2014, Jansson 2016), Denmark (Heinemann 2006, 2007, 2008, 2009a, 2011), the Netherlands (Caris-Verhallen et al. 1999), Germany (Sachweh 1998), South Africa (Makoni and Grainger 2002), the Philippines (Somera 1995, 1997), and Japan (Yamazaki et al. 2007, Backhaus 2009, 2010, 2011). In what follows, I will briefly outline the most salient characteristics that previous researchers have identified when exploring resident–staff interaction in institutional eldercare settings.

One of the key features of care institutions is that verbal communication itself tends to be rather scarce. In a comprehensive review of the literature on the topic, Grainger (2004b: 480) identifies a 'noticeable absence of talk between carers and residents' as one main theme in previous research. This echoes Lanceley (1985: 129), whose literature review from almost two decades earlier already identifies an 'overwhelming paucity of nurse–patient verbal interaction in the care of the elderly'.

Various quantitative studies have confirmed this tendency (see Grainger 2004b: 480–482). One of the more recent examples is Ward and his colleagues' (2008) research on dementia care in British nursing homes. Their study found that there was little direct contact between residents and staff, and that most of the interactions that did occur were shorter than five seconds. They summarise that 'silence is the dominant mode of caring encounters' (Ward et al. 2008: 636). Similar observations have been made in a study by Armstrong-Esther et al. (1994).

Lubinski (1988, 1995) has characterised institutional care as a 'communication impaired environment'. She stresses that this is not simply due to speech disorders on the part of the residents, but also a consequence of factors such as the physical setting (seating arrangements, background noise, etc.), poorly paid and educated staff working under severe time constraints, and low overall expectations with regard to the value of talking to one another. Citing similar constraints, Nussbaum (1991: 152) even calls the nursing home environment 'a place of potential "interactive starvation"'.

A second, partially overlapping theme is the task-oriented nature of care communication. As with many other forms of institutional interaction, the participants do not normally engage in talk for the sake of talk itself, but first and foremost do so in order to get things done. As Sachweh (2005: 47) summarises in a German primer on care communication, verbal interaction between residents and staff 'predominantly serves to announce, accompany, justify, or explain the necessary care activities'. Language in this context is seen as 'a tool to accomplish joint actions'.

Empirical studies support this observation. For instance, Wagnild and Manning (1985) in a study of bathing routines in geriatric long-term care facilities in Texas found that no less than half of the resident–staff interactions they examined either contained only task-oriented talk, or no talk at all. Grainger (2004b: 482–483) cites various other quantitative studies that demonstrate the predominance of the care tasks over more personal types of talk, a tendency she also finds reflected in her own data from a geriatric hospital in Wales (Grainger 1993a: 164–175, also 1993b: 251–252). Comparable observations have been made by Posenau (2014) in a recent study in a German care facility, who finds that the prime communicative aim in his data is the performance of the care activities. His analysis shows how this leaves its mark on various aspects of resident–staff communication, including the occurrence of openings without greetings, the low surface complexity of the care workers' utterances, and the disregard of residents' occasional resistance to suggested care procedures (Posenau 2014: 82, 149, 156).

This is not to say that the care tasks are the only topics residents and staff find themselves talking about. Previous researchers have identified a number of apparently non-task related modes of talk, varyingly referred to as 'time-out talk' (Fairhurst 1978, 1981), 'non-procedural' talk (Wagnild and Manning 1985), or 'social chit-chat' (Macleod-Clark 1982), among others. In care interaction, such instances of 'homileic discourse', as Ehlich and Rehbein (1980: 343) call it, do not normally occur in isolation (for an exception, see Marsden and Holmes 2014: 26), but coincide and concur with the task talk. This may result in a 'chatty mixture' of task and non-task oriented speech, as Gibb (1990: 16) observed in a study on bathing and showering routines in an Australian care facility.

A third common theme is the power asymmetries between residents and staff. As mentioned above, this is one of the general features of interaction in institutions. However, given the 'totality' of residential care, asymmetries can be considered more pronounced in such settings than in less total types of institutions such as schools or sport clubs. Hewison (1995) in his study of an English geriatric hospital has identified various ways the care workers' prerequisite to power becomes manifest in their speech. These include instructions and admonitions showing that 'the nurse is "in charge" and sets the parameters for what is and is not acceptable', continued persuasion when a resident has declined to follow the suggested course of actions, and the frequent use of terms of endearment to 'reinforce good behaviour'. Hewison also observes how the care workers frequently invoke institutional routines to justify their actions.

In her research in a German nursing home, Sachweh (2000) analyses the power differences between residents and staff with reference to Brown and Levinson's (1987, see section 4.2) politeness framework. She compiles a whole catalogue of poorly or non-redressed threats to a resident's face in the speech of the care workers that appear to be motivated by the power asymmetries of the institutional order: use of intimate second person pronoun address, use of pejorative expression and baby talk vocabulary, interruption and continuation of a resident's utterance in their stead, staff–staff talk about a resident in their presence, and unabated criticism of a resident's behaviour, among others (Sachweh 2000: 178–188).

In contrast to these findings, Marsden and Holmes (2014) in a study of two care facilities in New Zealand see an overall preference of solidarity over power. Their analysis shows that a majority of the interactions are characterised by 'warmth and friendliness' between caregivers and care recipients (Marsden and Holmes 2014: 31). This becomes manifest in their data in a variety of ways, including a recurring softening of the care workers' directives through lexical, syntactic, and prosodic devices, the reciprocal use of terms of endearment, and the occurrence of small talk dealing with topics pertaining to both the resident and the staff.

This relates to a last major theme, without which this literature review would surely remain incomplete: the occurrence of humour and joking. Grainger (2004a) in her data from Wales has identified humour as a viable strategy to negotiate power relations and deal with inherent face threats in institutional care. One of the examples she presents is from the bathing procedures, where joking is used to create a sense of familiarity that serves to 'legitimise the intimate help by a non-intimate other, to which the elderly adult is obliged to subject herself' (2004a: 48). In a similar vein, Marsden and Holmes (2014: 27–28) present several examples that show how 'humour may be especially useful in managing challenging, potentially embarrassing, or disagreeable situations'. Likewise, Davis et al. (2016: 57) emphasise that the use of 'gentle humor' in dementia care 'can mitigate tense situations that could otherwise elicit aggressive verbal or physical behaviors.'

Posenau (2014: 181) has observed how care workers in Germany use an intentionally exaggerated politeness register in order to play down the inherent asymmetry of their requests. Data from interactions in the Danish home help service even suggest that a care task such as changing diapers can be completed more quickly when the participants engage in some kind of joking or verbal play (Heinemann 2009a). As Lyman (1988: 97) summarises, based on observations in a US day care centre, humour thus 'can provide a real connection between people. It is an equalizer. When workers and patients intentionally, knowingly share humor, there is a tender moment between them'.

As can be seen, previous studies have determined a number of distinctive properties that characterise resident–staff interaction in eldercare settings throughout different cultural contexts. While the majority of researchers seem to take a comparatively critical view on these properties, there are also studies, most notably Marsden and Holmes (2014), which demonstrate that meaningful and satisfying communication can and does take place in the context of institutional eldercare. The next section takes a closer look at how the topic has been addressed by researchers in Japan.

2.3   Previous research in Japan

Against the backdrop of Japan's recent demographic developments, eldercare has become a topic of growing public and academic interest. Though communication makes up only a tiny part of the field as a whole, a fast growing number of academic publications suggest that the topic is increasingly being considered a subject worthy of scientific research.

A keyword search of the CiNii articles database (http://ci.nii.ac.jp/), which comprises a vast amount of Japanese academic publications from all scientific fields, may serve to illustrate this development. Figure 2.2 gives the total number

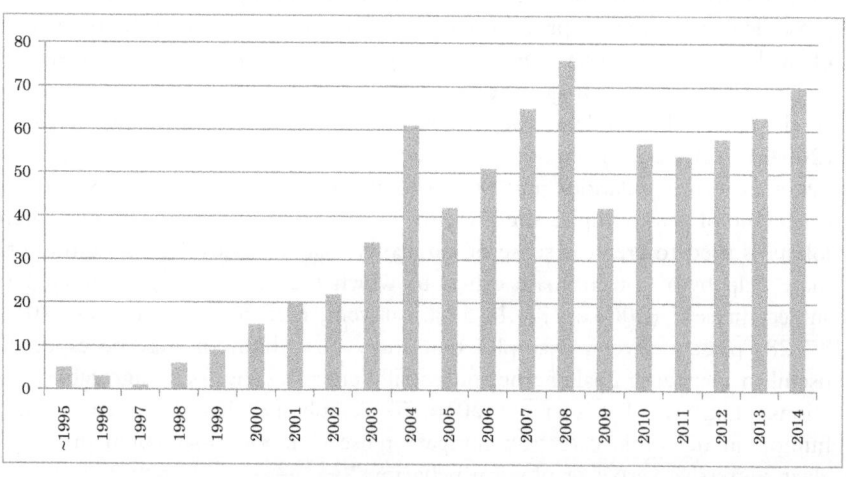

Figure 2.2 Academic publications containing the terms *kaigo* 'care' and *komyunikēshon* 'communication', 1980–2014.

Source: http://ci.nii.ac.jp/

of articles retrieved for the combined terms *kaigo* 'care' and *komyunikēshon* 'communication' between 1980 and 2014. As can be seen, only a handful of articles were published before 2000, the earliest being a 1986 study about the care of Parkinson patients (Shimanouchi 1986). After 2000, the number began quickly (though not quite steadily) rising, reaching an annual average output of between 60 and 70 publications as of 2014. Those most relevant to this study will now be briefly discussed.

One of the earliest studies of Japanese care communication was conducted by Amada (1999, cf. also 1997) in 1994. Based on field notes from four months of observation in the dementia ward of an unspecified eldercare facility, he observes that it is not necessarily the case that conversations between dementia patients are incoherent and chaotic, but that such features frequently result from the staff's task-oriented intrusion. In this respect, Amada observes that conversations between residents develop more easily in non-work spaces such as the lobby, whereas the dayroom and the cafeteria rarely produce any non-task related exchanges, and indeed little talk at all. Emphasising the issue of 'control', Amada (1999: 222) observes that routine work is commonly considered an end in itself in this type of 'management care' (*kanri kea*). He further criticises the frequent infantilisation of residents through inappropriate ways of speaking by the staff. Amada concludes his study with a few general suggestions to improve the situation for institutionalised dementia patients.

The topic of communication in dementia care has also been addressed by Naitō (2006), who worked with video recordings of dining room interactions in three care facilities in Aoyama, Nagano, and Kyoto prefectures. These recordings were played to other care professionals in order to identify problematic issues, with reference to Kitwood's (e.g., 1997, also see Ryan et al. 2005) concept of person-centred care. One commonly recognised problem was the performance of care actions that appeared detrimental to the residents' independence or were clearly rejected by them. In addition, the expert viewers criticised the high working tempo, which was found to produce many interactional mismatches. For example, it was frequently observed that when a care worker had announced an imminent action to a resident (e.g., aproning), the resident managed to respond to the announcement only after the action had already been accomplished. We will come back to the problem of tempo in chapters 7 and 8.

Ueda and her colleagues (2007) conducted a close-up study on interaction between care workers and a female resident in an unidentified Japanese group home. Based on video recordings of mealtimes, they examined how the care workers tried to train the slightly demented resident to properly chew with her new dentals. Ueda et al.'s careful observations show that despite the staff's recurrent efforts, there is no real improvement over time. Rather than re-learning the capacity to chew, the resident develops some quite remarkable skills to respond to the staff's instructions without having to change her way of chewing and choking at large. In this respect, the authors criticise the care workers for failing to notice some important details that were clearly visible on tape. On the other hand, they also observe that the resident shows little obvious resistance towards the staff's continuous directions and instructions, but, all in all, seems to be quite enjoying the attention devoted to her.

Developed out of a series of articles in a professional journal on nursing care, Hosoma's (2016) book *Kaigo suru karada* 'Bodies doing care' reflects on ten years of observations in institutional dementia care. Addressed at a larger, non-specialist audience, the book describes in great detail the author's 'discoveries' from everyday exchanges in various care facilities in western Japan. Emphasising the 'physicality' of social encounters, Hosoma is particularly interested in the non-verbal elements of care interaction and how they concur and interact with speech. Among many other things, he explores the common occurrence of 'heave-ho' expressions (*kakegoe*) and other interjections used to fine-tune and facilitate certain movements like swallowing or transferring (Hosoma 2016: 47–52, 59–61). As the analysis in chapter 6 will show, these elements also play a critical part in the present study. In addition, Hosoma (2016: 32) also takes a closer look at the use of ono-matopoetic expressions, emphasising that they have a vital timing function during care tasks and should therefore not be criticised as secondary baby talk.

Furuta and Horie (2011, 2014) have conducted a larger project on resident–staff interaction in a care facility in Hyogo prefecture. Their data consist of audio recordings from the bathing routines, including dressing and undressing the residents. One of the main topics they explore is the concurring usage of the plain and formal speech styles (see section 4.2). Their quantitative analysis shows that the interactions in the bathing room tend to contain more instances of formal language than those in the dressing room, which according to the authors may be a result of the scarcity of small talk during the bathing phase. In addition, Furuta and Horie identify various instances of positive politeness (Brown and Levinson 1987) in the speech of the care workers, including praise, joking, and the expression of empathy. Their analysis also includes some critical remarks on the power differences between residents and staff, and the latter's prerogative to determine the flow of the routines as a whole.

Originally aiming to provide adequate data for the development of care robots, Akiya and his colleagues (Akiya et al. 2006, 2007, 2009a, 2009b, Yamazaki et al. 2007) collected video data in various day care facilities across Japan. Their goal was to arrive at a more profound understanding of the interactional sensitivity such robots would need to acquire. Using conversation analytical methods, the study focuses on the problem of initiation activities in unstable multi-party settings such as the dayroom. The detailed analysis shows how the participants manage to establish a communication channel well in advance of any verbal exchange, display themselves as available, and commonly anticipate each other's actions through body signals and other non-verbal indications. The project is complemented by more experimental studies with student participants, who were instructed to act out specific types of care interactions (Akiya et al. 2006) or evaluate the interactive skills of a model robot (Akiya et al. 2009a). A more recent study reports on the development of a robot system intended to facilitate eye contact in multi-party interactions with and between wheelchair users (Suzuki et al. 2015).

In a separate project, Akiya (2008) uses video recordings from a day service facility in the Kansai area to examine the functioning of offers in initiating support activities. He applies Goffman's (1967) notion of facework and the conversation analytical concept of preference organisation (e.g., Atkinson and Heritage 1984: 53–56, Nofsinger 1991: 71–75), according to which offers are actions less socially risky than requests. Akiya presents several excerpts that show how care workers anticipate likely requests by the care recipients and offer support before being asked for it (also Akiya et al. 2008). Even when the offer is formulated in a more indirect way, the care recipients' prompt acceptance shows their appropriate construal of the care workers' intention. One excerpt explores the potential risks such offers may involve when turned down by a resident. As Akiya shows, this entails a long feedback loop of offers and rejects that reveals how each of the participants tries to implement their desired course of actions with minimal risks to the other's face.

Tachikawa's (2009, 2010, 2012, 2013, 2015) research was motivated by the advent of Indonesian and Philippine care workers and the perceived necessity to get a closer understanding of the basic linguistic requirements for communication in institutional care (similarly, Ōtani 2004). She uses data from a series of video recordings from care facilities in Toyama and Chiba prefectures. One of her early studies focuses on mealtime interactions. Tachikawa identifies a number of characteristics in the speech of the care workers, including a constant mixture of formal and plain speech styles, use of dialect, and the occurrence of baby talk. She also takes a closer look at the interplay of verbal and non-verbal actions, such as the care workers' frequent issuing of a backchannel token in reaction to a resident's physical movement (Tachikawa 2009).

In a later study, Tachikawa (2012) compiles a list of strategies the care workers employ to ensure a smooth performance of the care tasks. These include use of referent and addressee honorifics (see sections 4.2 and 4.3), preference of requests over directives, use of the modifying adverb *chotto* 'just, a little', and other negative politeness features. She also identifies instances of positive politeness such as the use of hortative forms (see section 5.1) and other relatively intimate ways of speaking that serve to evoke a family relationship and thus fulfil an important function in establishing rapport (Tachikawa 2012: 94). With respect to the education of foreign care workers, Tachikawa (2015: 70) concludes that a sufficient command of Japanese appears to be indispensable for providing good care. She emphasises that this goes far beyond mere knowledge of technical terms, but also requires substantial interactional skills (Tachikawa 2012: 94).

As part of a larger project on communication in the welfare sector, Kitamoto (2006, 2007: 98–118) collected data in a nursing home in Tokyo. She made video recordings of three care workers throughout each one's daytime shift. The transcripts were analysed using word mining software. Zooming in on the number of turns in the speech of the care workers, Kitamoto shows that though there are considerable individual differences with respect to the total amount of talk, the ratio between delivered and 'received' speech is relatively similar for all three care workers.

In a second step, Kitamoto identifies a basic micro structure that is recognisable in a large number of the staff–resident interactions. Discussing three excerpts in detail, she exemplifies how such interactions normally start with some sort of opening, continue with a phase of 'information collection' and physical support, and are concluded with a recognisable closing exchange. The analysis is complemented by a list of the most frequent vocabulary items in the opening and closing phases of the data.

Onoda (2007, 2008, 2009, 2010, 2011, 2013, 2014) has examined communication between care workers and care recipients in a number of Japanese home help settings. Working with audio recordings made in the Chūbu region, he analyses the occurrence of talk in general, as well as its narrative structure and most common topics. He makes a basic distinction between topics directly related to the running care task and topics that develop independent of it. For example, in one of his earlier studies, he found that 80% of the recording time was filled with talk, with a relatively balanced speech participation of home helper and care recipient. In terms of contents, 66% of all talk was not directly related to the task, and frequently not related to care in general (Onoda 2007). In a more recent paper, Onoda (2014) explores how such instances of non-task talk frequently develop out of talk about a running task or are triggered by physical items in the environment, which are easily turned into conversational material.

Other issues Onoda's research deals with are conflicts in interactions between care recipient and care manager (Onoda 2009), overall differences in interactions with home helpers as compared to interactions with care managers (Onoda 2008, 2010), and the concurrence of two different 'expression styles' (*hyōgen yōshiki*) that may help explain misunderstandings and the seeming lack of coherence in the speech of care recipients (Onoda 2013). Incidentally, Onoda has also been in charge of a recent 'care and communication' (*kaigo to kotoba*) column in the Japanese journal *Nihongogaku* (Onoda 2016a, 2016b, 2016c, 2016d), which testifies to the growing importance of the topic in general.

Interaction in home help care is also dealt with in a paper by Koike (2000), in which she reflects on her long-term experiences with seven consecutive care professionals looking after her mother. Based on daily observations, Koike critically explores the performance of each care worker with respect to their way of speaking, their technical skills, their impression on the care recipient, and various other aspects. She notices substantial differences in the communication style of each care worker, including use of plain or formal speech style, directive speech, use of dialect, and talkativeness, among others.

Another common way previous researchers have approached the topic of communication in Japanese eldercare is through a systematic coding of activities over longer stretches of time. For example, Matsunaga and Iseki (2004) studied the daily interaction of 19 dementia patients in an unspecified care facility. They took notes of the residents' verbal and non-verbal exchanges in one-minute intervals and coded their emotions as conveyed through facial expression, gestures, tone of voice, and a number of other features. They found that the residents on average spent over 70% of the day without being engaged in any form of communication. Though it proved difficult to assess the residents' emotional state at these non-interactional points in time, the analysis reveals that they showed mostly positive feelings when being part of a communicative exchange. Similar methods of coding have been applied by Furukawa et al. (2002), Suzuki et al. (2002), Komatsu et al. (2003), Kaneda (2005), and Sugiyama et al. (2008). The latter's study in a dementia care facility in Tokyo also shows a statistically significant correlation between a resident's self-reported wellbeing and the occurrence of everyday conversation.

Yet another line of research is experimental studies. One example is Yoshikawa and his colleagues' work with audio recordings of small-group interactions in open spaces of various dementia care facilities in the Tohoku region. Two types of care workers were involved: While one group was doing ordinary shift work, the second group was released from all tasks other than engaging in communication with the residents. Quantitative analysis of the transcripts shows that conversations involving a care worker exclusively dedicated to talking with the residents were both more lively (higher number of turns, more overlaps, etc.) and more coherent (fewer utterances out of context) than conversations with a care worker on an ordinary shift. This suggests that the presence of a 'talk-only' care worker, if affordable, can have a highly positive effect on the quality of communication in dementia care (Yoshikawa et al. 2004).

Yoshikawa and his research team also experimentally explore the topics of speech accommodation (Yoshikawa et al. 2005) and patronising talk (Yoshikawa and Sugai 2005). Using a similar approach, Takemura and collaborators (1999) tested the long-term effects of a predominantly conversational speech mode as opposed to a more activity-driven way of speaking. They found that the former had a much more favourable influence on institutional dementia patients. In other experiments, Goto and her colleagues (2010) paired day care users with Korean exchange students in order to identify potential communication difficulties for non-native caregivers, while Kim and his colleagues (2000) examined the effects of an electronic communication system on a Japanese dementia patient in an unspecified day care centre.

Finally, a considerable number of researchers have approached Japanese care communication through questionnaire studies or interviews. An early example is Suzuki (2001), who explored the communicative skills of several hundred care professionals in the Tohoku region by presenting them with a questionnaire of 33 items for self-evaluation on basic and more specified skills in verbal interaction with care recipients. Similar studies, some slightly different in scope, have been made by Komatsu (2005), Matsuyama (2006), Yamada and Nishida (2007), Yoshida (2007), Owada and Kagaya (2008), Watanabe (2008), Yokoi (2009), Yoshitomi (2009), Harada (2014), Tanaka (2014), and Kambe (2015). Research based on interviews with caregivers was done by Shibuya and colleagues (2008), who focus on communication problems in dementia care, as well as Yasutome (2009) and Tachikawa (2011), both of whom deal with the topic of communication with foreign caregivers.

Taken together, the above overview shows that communication in eldercare is a topic of growing interest in Japan's rapidly ageing society. Since the beginning of the new century, researchers from diverse fields and with differing perspectives and motivations have contributed a greater number of empirical studies. Some use conversation analytical approaches to take a fine-grained look at the interactional micro-level, while others work more quantitatively and/or experimentally to capture and compare interactional features in 'hard numbers'. Yet another group of researchers choose social psychological approaches by collecting data through interviews or questionnaire surveys with caring staff.

In comparison with research outside Japan, as discussed in the previous section, it is worthwhile noting that many of the observations made by Japanese researchers concur with findings from studies elsewhere. These include the overall scarcity of communication in eldercare settings (Amada 1999, Matsunaga and Iseki 2004, but see also Onoda 2007), the influence of the care tasks on the verbal interaction (Yoshikawa et al. 2004, Naitō 2006, Onoda 2014), power differences (Fukada 2009, Furuta and Horie 2011) and the infantilisation of residents through patronising talk (Amada 1999, Yoshikawa and Sugai 2005, Tachikawa 2009, but see also Hosoma 2016: 32), and use of various politeness features to circumvent or abate possible face threats (Koike 2000, Furuta and Horie 2011, Tachikawa 2012). From an applied perspective, many of the studies further recognise the importance of talk in itself, stressing that it must be considered one key element in providing satisfactory care (Matsunaga and Iseki 2004, Yoshikawa et al. 2004, Naitō 2006).

What is – to some extent at least – Japan-specific about the literature discussed in this section is that a larger part of the more recent studies seem to be motivated by current socio- and techno-political developments in the Japanese care sector.

Most noteworthy in this respect is the advent of foreign care workers. Even though less than 500 applicants from EPA countries have passed the required state exam so far (Matsukawa and Morimoto 2016), their presence has become a big social issue in a society that used to define itself as culturally homogeneous, non-immigrant, and monolingual (Lie 2000, Noguchi 2001, also see Świtek 2014). The 'foreign element' in care has entailed an increased interest in care communication as such, which has been the main drive for a greater number of the studies discussed in this section.

The heightened consciousness of foreign care workers is also reflected in a 2009 publication of a little Japanese–English glossary of care language that explicitly addresses a non-Japanese workforce (JFKC 2009). More recently, and perhaps more to the point, a book with a similar intent was published that 'translates' difficult care lingo into more easily understandable Japanese, also known as *yasashii Nihongo* (Endō and Saegusa 2015).

A second factor that has triggered researchers' (and research funders') interest is the growing use of robots and robotic devices in care contexts and their future potential as non-human workforce. Here, too, a closer understanding of (human–human) care interaction is vital for further technological developments. With respect to public opinion towards these trends, it is perhaps interesting to note that according to a recent (non-representative) newspaper survey, care work ranked highest among a number of tasks (warfare, medicine, cooking, love) that people wish to see transferred to robots (Asahi Shimbun 2015).

Whatever stance one may take towards these trends, they have certainly had their share in raising scientific interest in care communication as a topic of crucial importance to the world's oldest and most quickly ageing society.

3   Data and methodology

The aim of this chapter is to give a basic outline of the empirical research conducted for this project. We start with a brief introduction to the research setting under observation, followed by a few remarks on how the data were recorded, documented, selected, and prepared for analysis. The second section more closely describes the data sample on which the analysis in the subsequent chapters is based. It also introduces the participants involved and the activities they are commonly engaged in. In addition, the compilation of the final sample of interactions is described. The third section presents the research question of this study and the methods used to address it. The chapter closes with a few critical reflections on methodological issues to be taken into account.

3.1   Data collection

A pilot study to this project was conducted in spring 2007 in a residential care facility in central Tokyo. After getting in touch with the institution via an acquaintance, I was allowed to accompany the care workers for two weeks and assist with small tasks such as feeding and dressing the residents. This made me gain some first insights into the everyday life of institutional care in Japan, and some of its communicative characteristics (see Backhaus 2009). Unfortunately, it was not possible to gain permission for recordings, so I had to rely entirely on field notes. This was the main reason why I decided to look for another environment to continue my research.

   The place to which I was finally granted admission is a care facility situated at the northern outskirts of the Tokyo Metropolitan region. Edogawa Care, as I will refer to it here, is administratively classified as a geriatric health care facility, or *kaigo rōjin hoken shisetsu*. Facilities of this type were established after a 1986 revision of the Law for Health Care of the Elderly (*rōjin hoken-hō*). They provide both essential medical care and everyday life support, with the ultimate goal of preparing their users for a life back home. In reality, however, they frequently function as 'transit facilities' (*tsūkai shisetsu*) (Ōta and Miyoshi 2005: 132) or 'fixed-term residential facilities' (*kikantsuki no nyūsho shisetu*) (Yuki 2008: 38) for people looking for long-time residential care. There are more than 4,100 geriatric health care facilities nationwide, accommodating a total of over 350,000 monthly users (MHLW 2016b).

The Edogawa Care facility has three floors. The ground floor is used as a day care facility for outpatients; the two upper floors are residential. The second floor is designed for residents suffering from dementia, while the third floor mainly accommodates users without such symptoms. An approximate number of 50 residents live on each of the two upper floors, mostly in four-bed rooms. In line with common practice in Japanese healthcare settings, each bed is visually separable from the rest of the room with a bed curtain. All rooms are equipped with a toilet/bathroom. In addition, each floor has one large community bathing space that is used twice a week by all residents. In the centre of each floor is a large dayroom, where the meals are served and various recreational and rehabilitation activities are conducted. Residents are expected to eat in the dayroom and spend most of the day time there.

After two weeks of participant observations on all three floors, I decided to focus on the morning care activities on the third floor. I did so because these turned out to be one of the few occasions where longer stretches of relatively stable dyadic resident–staff interactions would occur. This is partly in line with Grainger (1993a: 62), who in her study in a Welsh care facility observed that 'nurse-patient interaction takes place almost exclusively during care routines'. Similar approaches with focus on the morning care have been taken by Gibb (1990), Sachweh (2000), Wadensten (2005), Posenau (2014), and Jansson (2016).

Actions performed during the morning care include waking up the residents and getting them out of bed, washing and dressing them, supporting them with going to the toilet, and accompanying them to the dayroom. In line with common practice in Japan, the largest part of the morning care in Edogawa Care is done by the two care workers on night shift. The activities start around 4:30 in the morning and are largely completed by 7:00, when an additional care worker from the early daytime shift (*hayaban*) arrives. Breakfast is served at 7:30; the ordinary day shift (*nikkin*) starts at 8:30.

The data were recorded during a period of six weeks in October and November 2007. On each recording day, one of the two care workers from the night shift would attach a small pin microphone to the collar of their jacket or shirt, which was connected to a portable digital recording device in their pocket. This procedure allowed for uninterrupted recordings throughout the whole of one care worker's interactions during the morning care activities, normally from after 4:30 to around 6:30. Either me or a Japanese colleague was present during the recordings. In order to be minimally intrusive, we did not follow the care workers into the residents' rooms, but took notes about each recorded care worker's morning care 'route' from some distance.

We recorded on a total of 18 working days featuring nine different care workers. The total recording time is about 38 hours, with an approximate average length of 110 minutes per day. Directly after each recording, we compared the audio data with our notes from that day and created an overview of the main flow of activities, in intervals of 15 seconds. These activity logs, as they will subsequently be referred to, were to provide us with a basic idea about what a care worker was doing when and with whom. Particularly in view of the non-availability of video date, this turned out to be extremely helpful for the later analysis.

I eventually decided to focus on two recordings of each care worker, which means that 'third' recordings and care workers with only one recording were discarded. This reduced the number of days to 12. The recordings of these days were more closely examined with respect to interactions that would qualify as morning care in a narrower sense. In order to keep the data comparable, only those interactions were analysed that clearly mark the start of a morning care exchange and continue until the care worker and the resident first 'part ways' (excluding a few cases where a care worker temporarily left to fetch something but directly returned). This means that chance encounters in the hallway or the dayroom, as well as all 'resumed' activities, even if clearly part of the morning care, were excluded from the analysis. A few critical reflections on this way of cutting up the data are given in section 3.3.

In some cases, the interactions of the sample are not completely dyadic but involve brief sequences that feature a third or fourth person: a resident from the same room, residents moving through the hallway, a resident on nurse call, another care worker or, occasionally, one of the two researchers (though we were doing our best to stay aloof). However, such instances were usually very short and did not seem to have a lasting effect on the interactional flow. The analysis of the data concentrates on the two 'protagonists' of an interaction: one care worker and one resident as they work their way through the morning care routines.

3.2   The sample

The sample thus compiled consists of 107 (mostly) dyadic resident–staff interactions. The data include four female and two male care workers. All of them were in their late 20s or early 30s, with an average age of 28 years. The residents' average age by the time of the survey was 77 years. A total of 25 persons were involved, 14 female and 11 male residents. The gender pairings of the interactions are summarised in Table 3.1.

Table 3.1 Gender pairings of the interactions

Staff	*Resident*	
Female	Female	43
Female	Male	30
Male	Female	19
Male	Male	15
		107

The overall predominance of female participants roughly reflects the basic gender structure in Edogawa Care, where women make up a majority both in the group of the care workers and in the group of the residents. Although this was not specifically intended, it also concurs with the gender bias in Japanese eldercare in general (Coulmas 2007: 65). All participants were native speakers of Japanese, mostly from the Kanto region that includes the larger capital area.

All 107 interactions start in a resident's room. In a few cases, the care worker arrives on scene after being called by the resident via the intercom system, but the majority of exchanges start without a previous nurse call. When the care worker enters, the residents are usually still in bed. After the basic care activities have been performed (getting out of bed, diaper change/intimate care, parts of the dressing), the residents are normally accompanied by the care workers to the toilet at the entrance area of the room. If that toilet is occupied, the care worker chooses a toilet from one of the adjacent rooms. From the toilet, where often parts of the dressing are continued, most of the residents will later be accompanied through the hallway to the washing section in the dayroom, where they are asked to brush their teeth or put in their dentals, wash their face, and comb their hair. When they are finished, they are wheeled to their customary table in the dayroom, where they will be served tea, chat with other residents, watch TV on one of the two flat screens in the room, or just sit.

In the majority of cases, the care worker leaves the resident at the toilet to take up some other task until the resident calls via intercom. This means that most of the 107 interactions of the sample end at the toilet. In other cases, an interaction may come to a close while the participants are still in the resident's room. This usually happens with relatively independent residents who can go to the toilet by themselves. An in-room closing may also occur when a care worker suspends the morning care activities to attend to a nurse call or some other urgent matter. Alternatively, a resident sometimes returns with a care worker to her or his room after finishing toilet use, though these are rather exceptional cases.

As can be seen in Table 3.2, only a small number of the exchanges continue without interruption until the resident's arrival in the dayroom. With regard to the analysis of the data, this means that the beginning of the recorded interactions in most of the cases marks the beginning of the morning care activities as such. By contrast, the end of an interaction only rarely coincides with the actual end of the morning care, but usually precedes it.

Table 3.2 Places and place shifts

Places of interaction	
Room only	23
Room > toilet	67
Room > toilet > hallway/dayroom	8
Room > hallway/dayroom	7
Room > toilet > room	2
	107

The average length of the interactions is 4 minutes and 20 seconds. The shortest interaction takes about one minute (#49), which seems sufficient for a care worker to get a resident out of bed and to the toilet. By contrast, the longest interaction of the sample is over 12 minutes. It features a care worker and a resident in the resident's room, the toilet, the hallway, and finally the washing section in the dayroom (#85). The standard deviation is 2 minutes, 19 seconds.

Regarding the relatively huge differences in the length of the interactions, one general observation is that the time a care worker spends 'on' a resident is not determined by the amount of talk the participants want to exchange, but by the amount of work that needs to be done. That is why the end of an interaction always falls together with the end (or temporary suspension) of a task. This point, to which we will come back during the analysis, is in line with observations in previous research on communication in institutional eldercare (e.g., Sachweh 2000: 74).

All 107 interactions were transcribed using ELAN, an annotation program developed at the Max Planck Institute for Psycholinguistics (https://tla.mpi.nl/tools/tla-tools/elan/). As described in the introduction, transcription largely follows Jefferson's conventions (Atkinson and Heritage 1984: ix–xvi, Jefferson 2004), a list of which is attached in Appendix 1. Japanese was transcribed using Kanji and Kana, but is romanised in the excerpts of this book. In order to make the data analysable with concordance software, the transcripts were later tokenised with ChaSen (http://chasen-legacy.osdn.jp/). The concordancer used was AntConc (http://www.laurenceanthony.net/software/antconc/).

3.3   Research question and methodological considerations

The main motivation for this research is to get a better overall understanding about the nature of communication in Japanese institutional eldercare settings. Thus the research question that guides the analysis has been intentionally kept broad: What are the basic characteristics of resident–staff interaction during the morning care activities in Edogawa Care?

To address this question, I apply a mixture of methods that could best be located within the field of interactional sociolinguistics (e.g., Tannen 1992, Berenz 2001, Bailey 2008). I take advantage of the framework of conversation analysis (CA), which provides a sophisticated set of analytical tools to capture and explore naturally occurring interactions in both institutional and non-institutional contexts. CA is an inductive approach that starts out with 'unmotivated looking' at single cases from which larger principles can be derived. One of the main tenets of CA is the orderliness of talk in interaction and how such orderliness is produced by the participants on a turn-by-turn basis (e.g., Liddicoat 2007, Hutchby and Wooffitt 2008, Garcia 2013). It is the detection of such micro-level orderliness that motivates large parts of the analysis in the subsequent chapters.

I also use concepts from variationist sociolinguistics where feasible, relating communication patterns as they appear in the interaction to social variables such as gender and institutional role (e.g., Coupland and Jaworski 1997: 163–167, Macaulay 2005). A third field I borrow from is corpus linguistics, which provides various helpful tools for exploring large amounts of data. While the main focus of my analysis is on the micro structure of the interactions, I found a corpus analytical approach beneficial in that it allows for occasional looks at the data from a bird's eye perspective.

Finally, I had the chance to present some of the intermediate findings of my research to the staff at Edogawa Care in three 'study sessions' (*benkyōkai*) held in July 2010, 2012, and 2014. Where feasible, I triangulate my interpretations of the data with this first-hand feedback from the participants. This ethnographic supplement is particularly important in view of the fact that I am a cultural outsider to the research setting, which entails the advantage of a fresh perspective, but, needless to say, also involves certain risks of getting things wrong, or not getting them at all.

One serious methodological problem that cannot go unaddressed is the non-availability of video data. Whereas audio recordings have the advantage of being easier to collect in a minimally intrusive way, it has become increasingly commonsensical in CA and related fields to work with video data (see, e.g., the seminal studies by Goodwin 1984, Heath 1986). Researchers today agree that a large part of talk in interactions relies on non-verbal elements such as gaze, body posture, and gestures – information that remains inaccessible if only audio data are available. As I was to realise later on, this 'tapping in the dark' will necessarily leave large parts of the analysis somewhat hanging in the air. Unfortunately, it was impractical to get permission for video recordings in this very intimate setting, so faced with the choice of having no data or only 'invisible' data, I went for the latter option.

Another issue is the possible interference of the observer(s) on the flow of the interactions. As with all types of data that were collected after informing and receiving consent from the participants, it can never be ruled out that the fact of being recorded in itself might have some effect on the recorded behaviour. However, my overall impression was that the participants did not substantially deviate from their usual way of doing things as I had observed it prior to the recordings. In addition, some of the care workers later commented that they were so busy with their work that after a few minutes they had entirely forgotten they were being taped. This is in line with Skovdahl et al.'s (2003: 897) experiences in a Swedish care facility, who also cite a number of similar examples from previous research.

On a personal note, I may add that I have some experience with being a subject of recording myself. Though these were entirely unrelated projects, this view from the 'other side of the microphone' served to assure me that the overall consciousness about being recorded while working is negligibly low. And even if the fact of being taped should have some impact on the linguistic performance, I agree with Garcia's (2013: 32) view that the resulting changes are 'more likely to be in the content of the conversation than in the procedures used to conduct it'. It is on the latter that this study is focused.

A final methodological problem is the 'vivisection' of a day's recording into a somewhat arbitrary number of smaller units. As described above, this was mainly done for practical reasons, and proved quite helpful for getting a grip on the data and establishing some comparability. However, it must not be forgotten that these little morning care 'bites' that we end up analysing do not and did not exist in isolation. For the participants, they are but one instance in a long line of previous and subsequent encounters on this day and other days. For example, as the morning care is done by the night shift, the analysed interactions in many cases are not really the first encounter between resident and care worker on that day. Similarly, the participants know that the 'end' of an interaction rarely coincides with the last encounter they are going to have with each other before the care worker goes off shift. Care must be taken that this larger context is sufficiently taken into account. I have tried to do so by closely re-reading the activity log of each selected survey day to keep track of the flow of events as a whole. However, these logs are merely the tip of an iceberg, the main part of which must remain invisible to the observer's eye.

Despite these limitations, I believe that the 107 morning interactions collected for this study provide a workable empirical basis for exploring the main inter-actional characteristics in the setting under observation. We start with a closer look at the occurrence of honorifics.

4 Honorifics

Honorifics can be defined as 'special linguistic forms that are used as signs of deference toward the nominal referents or the addressee' (Shibatani 2001: 552) of a communicative encounter. In contrast to many western languages, Japanese is known as a language with a sophisticated grammatical system of such forms. It has a large inventory of lexical and morphosyntactic devices to express deference towards both the referent and the addressee of a speech event, as well as various other contextual features.

This chapter takes a first look at the occurrence of honorifics in the 107 morning care interactions of the data. The chief aim is to introduce the main types of Japanese honorifics and give a rudimentary overview of their usage in Edogawa Care. We start with one basic type of honorific: terms of address. The analysis explores the most common terms residents and staff use to call each other during the morning care interactions and examines the main differences between the two groups. After that, we examine the speech level of the interactions, which is arguably the most complex aspect of Japanese honorifics. The third section focuses on referent honorifics. It provides an overview of the most common types of humbling, exalting, and beautifying forms, and how they interact with each other and with other honorific levels.

The analysis in this chapter is not predominantly concerned with the topic of politeness. Research since the late 1990s has increasingly propagated a move away from formal approaches and called for a conceptualising of politeness as a problem that, if at all, can be properly understood only in interaction. In line with this 'discursive turn' (Haugh 2007: 302), the study of honorifics, formal by definition, has gone somewhat out of fashion. While I explicitly welcome most recent trends in this direction, I believe that a focused analysis of honorifics will have some value in its own right for the present research purpose. We will come back to the topic of politeness and its thorny relationship with honorifics in the general discussion in chapter 8.

4.1 Terms of address

Address as a technical term refers to 'a speaker's linguistic reference to his/her collocutor(s)' (Braun 1988: 7). The way people call each other is one of the most salient interfaces between language and society, as it almost inevitably indexes different degrees of formality, interpersonal relationships, and speaker identities. Terms of address thus form part of the core variables in early sociolinguistic research.

A seminal paper on the topic was Brown and Gilman's (1960) analysis of pronoun usage in various western societies, for which they identified a common distinction between a formal 'V address', usually by means of a second person plural pronoun, and a more informal 'T address' in second person singular. Languages that do not (or no longer) have a distinctive pronominal address system regularly use nominal devices to express such differences. Thus a subsequent paper by Brown and Ford (1961) identified two main address forms in American English: first name (FN) and (title plus) last name (LN) address. Subsequent accounts of the situation in English were provided by Ervin-Tripp (1972), Hook (1984), Leech (1999), and Murray (2002). The development in various other European languages is explored in Clyne et al. (2009) and Norrby and Wide (2015).

A basic distinction can be made between referential and vocative address. While the former factually means speaking about someone who also happens to be the addressee of an utterance, the latter is used 'for calling out and attracting or maintaining the addressee's attention' (Daniel and Spencer 2009: 626). Zwicky (1974: 787), who was among the first to deal with this distinction in English, presents the following examples: In 'You should hand me those forceps', the address term 'you' is used referentially, whereas in 'You, hand me those forceps', it occurs as a vocative. Braun (1988: 11) makes a similar distinction between bound (= referential) and free (= vocative) address forms. She observes that there appears to be an overall tendency for pronominal forms to be used mainly in referential address, whereas vocative address commonly relies on nominal forms. However, there are some rather pronounced cross-linguistic differences with respect to what linguistic form can be used in which of the two functions, a point we will come back to in the course of the discussion.

Various previous studies have examined the use of address terms in institutional interaction. Research is available from a large number of (mostly western) contexts, including workplace settings (Slobin et al. 1968, Hartmann 1972, Warren 2006, Clyne et al. 2009: 100–107), service encounters (Clyne et al. 2009: 107–114, Félix-Brasdefer 2015: 204–226, Isosävi and Lappalainen 2015, Norrby et al. 2015, Placencia 2015), doctor–patient interaction (Henzl 1989: 88–89), courtroom hearings (Jacquemet 1994), TV and radio interviews (McCarthy and O'Keeffe 2003, Rendle-Short 2007, Vismans 2015), political debates (Jaworski and Galasiński 2000, Ilie 2010), team sports (Wilson 2010), and various academic settings (Dickey 1997, Belz and Kinginger 2003, Clyne et al. 2009: 94–100, Formentelli 2009). One overarching point these studies make is that the choice of address terms is not merely reflective of social relationships, but can play an important part in fine-tuning and manipulating these very relationships.

An early empirical study about terms of address in institutional eldercare was conducted by Wagnild and Manning (1985). In their research on bathing routines in geriatric long-term care facilities in Texas, they found that while the care workers addressed the majority of the residents by their last name, there were also instances of first name address and various terms of endearments. This was in stark contrast to the corresponding address behaviour by the residents, who hardly ever called the staff directly by name. Looking more closely into this matter in follow-up interviews, Wagnild and Manning found that only 15% of the residents happened to know the name of the nurse that had attended to them. This is an illustrative example of how institutionally defined differences in access to knowledge may affect the linguistic interaction, as mentioned in chapter 2.

A comparable problem has been identified by Sachweh (2000: 242–249) in a study in German nursing homes. Her analysis shows that the residents in many cases appeared not to know the last name of the care workers and, consequently, either had to use their first name or rely on alternative ways of address such as *Schwester* 'nurse'. These findings are largely in line with Posenau's (2014: 66–77) observations in two other German care facilities, though the two studies differ with respect to the residents' use of pronominal address. Whereas in Sachweh's data, the V address pronoun *Sie* was the most common choice, the residents in Posenau's study, most of whom suffered from more severe degrees of dementia, normally addressed the care workers with the more informal *du*. A general discussion of the use of *du* and *Sie* in German eldercare is given by Meißner (2005).

Before turning to the data of the present study, a few general comments about Japanese terms of address are in order, as there are various differences compared to English and other western languages. First, pronouns are rarely used as terms of address. The main rule of thumb, as concisely summarised by McClure (2000: 234), is 'to avoid them completely in very polite conversation, and to avoid them as much as possible everywhere else'. Instead, conversational partners are commonly called by their (first or last) name, normally with the person honorific suffix *-san* attached. In addition, there is a large number of address terms to express professional, family, or other role relationships (e.g., Takenoya 2003: 18–23, Kitayama 2013). Likely the most common way of person reference though is zero anaphora, that is, no explicit address form at all. As Japanese syntax almost unrestrictedly allows for noun phrase ellipsis, the 'you' part of an utterance does not have to be linguistically encoded but can be omitted whenever retrievable from context (e.g., Yamaguchi 2007: 113–117, Iwasaki 2013: 279–282).

With respect to the distinction between vocative and referential address, the greatest difference between English and Japanese is that while in English, referential use of address terms is largely confined to pronouns, in Japanese this can just as well be done by nominal forms. Thus, the 'you' in both of Zwicky's aforementioned example sentences in Japanese could easily be replaced by the addressee's last name (LN), or another nominal term of address. So when asking for the said tool, not only 'LN-*san*, hand me those forceps' but also 'LN-*san* should hand me those forceps' would be possible in Japanese (e.g., Ide 1982: 358, Länsisalmi 2001: 139).

Another noteworthy feature of Japanese address terms is what Braun (1988: 9) has called the 'fictive use of kinship terms'. In Japan, it is quite normal to address a person by using a term denoting a family relationship that does not actually apply (e.g., Niyekawa 1991: 104, Traphagan 2000: 76–77, Bu 2004). This phenomenon is also reported to occur in institutional eldercare (see, e.g., Bethel 1992a: 114, Kinoshita and Kiefer 1992: 183), where the potentially harmful effects of this way of address have been discussed within the wider context of Hummert and Ryan's (1996) framework of patronising talk (e.g., Usami 1997, 1999, Usami and Endō 1997). As a result, attempts have been made in recent years to ban terms such as *ojii-san* 'gran' and *obaa-chan* 'granny' from geriatric hospital wards and eldercare institutions (see Backhaus 2008: 458–460).

Informed by previous research, the analysis in this section looks at the use of address terms from two complementary angles: (1) how the care workers address the residents, and (2) how the residents address the care workers. To this end, all 107 interactions were first searched for the occurrence of address terms, both in vocative and in referential function, as used by the two main participants to refer to each other. All items that were identified in an interaction were classified with respect to resident vs. staff usage and address term type.

4.1.1   Staff vs. residents

The overall occurrence of address terms as used by the care workers in each of the 107 interactions is summarised in Table 4.1. Leaving aside for a moment the 23 cases that do not contain an address term by the care worker involved, we can see that there are two main ways the staff in Edogawa Care address the residents. The most frequent choice is a resident's last name (LN) plus honorific -*san*, used in 75% of the relevant interactions. Another common way of addressing a resident is using her or his first name (FN), again with -*san*. This more intimate address is chosen by the care workers in 23% of the cases.

Only two cases do not completely fit into the LN/FN pattern. The first one is an exchange in which a care worker first calls a resident FN-*san*, in the course

Table 4.1 Terms of address used by the care workers

Term of address	Number of interactions
LN-*san*	63 (75%)
FN-*san*	19 (23%)
LN-*san* + FN-*san*	1 (1%)
LN-*san* + *okaa-san*	1 (1%)
	84 (100%)

Note: Of the 107 interactions, 23 did not contain address terms by the care workers.

of the interaction shifts to LN-*san*, and in closing moves back to the FN-*san* address (#101). A similar case is discussed by Sachweh (2003: 156–157). However, this is the only example in the data where a shift between first name and last name address occurs within one interaction, suggesting that there is generally little variation in the way a care worker calls a resident during the morning care.

And then there is in fact one interaction in which a care worker addresses a resident by a kinship term. The circumstances are as follows: The resident has been in a miserable mood since she got up, and has started crying briefly after that. The care worker throughout the interaction makes numerous and increasingly desperate attempts to cheer her up. It is during this situation of high emotional distress that she addresses the resident two times using the term *okaa-san* 'mother' when telling her that there is no need to cry. The fact that this is the only instance in the sample where a resident is addressed this way suggests that the fictive use of kinship terms is no common practice in Edogawa Care. Of further note is that the care worker uses the relatively neutral term *okaa-san* rather than the more age indicative *obaa-san* 'grandma' or the hyper-coristic *obaa-chan* 'granny', which are the terms that have been in the centre of criticism.

Moving on with the analysis, we will now focus on the way each of the 23 residents is addressed individually by the care workers across the interactions. A closer look reveals that the choice between first name and last name is relatively clearly determined. Most residents are consistently called either FN-*san* (n = 4) or LN-*san* (n = 16) by all care workers. Only three residents are addressed by some staff members by last name while others use their first name. This finding suggests that there is some implicit understanding among the staff as to how a given resident should be addressed.

One factor that seems to influence the care workers' choice between FN and LN address is a resident's gender. As can be seen in Table 4.2, male residents are not usually addressed by their first name, for which there is only one exception in the data. In all other cases where FN address occurs, the addressee is a woman. In total, no less than 6 of the 14 female residents in the sample are called at least by some of the care workers by their first name. Though the overall number of cases is rather small, it seems that reservations to use a resident's first name are much less pronounced when talking to a woman than when talking to a man. This is largely in line with previous observations on

Table 4.2 Terms of address vs. resident's gender

Residents called	Male	Female	Total
Only LN-*san*	8	8	16
Only FN-*san*	1	3	4
LN-*san* or FN-*san*		3	3
	9	14	23

Table 4.3 Interactions containing address terms, residents vs. staff

Term of address	Residents to staff	Staff to residents
Not used	96 (89.7%)	23 (21.5%)
Used	11 (10.3%)	84 (78.5%)
Total	**107 (100%)**	

gender differences in terms of address usage in other contexts (see Holmes 1995: 145–149 for an overview).

If we now take a comparative look at how the residents address the staff, the most important point to note is that in the overall majority of cases, they do not address them at all. As Table 4.3 shows, there are only 11 interactions (12.6%) in which a resident directly refers to a care worker by an address term. This is in stark contrast to the care workers' speech, added to Table 4.3 for ease of comparison, which, as we have seen, in the large majority of the interactions contains at least one address term towards the person spoken to.

Echoing previous research, this asymmetry in the address behaviour of the two groups can best be explained by the institutional setting and the differences in the participants' access to knowledge (Wagnild and Manning 1985, Sachweh 2000). As to the care workers, it is part of their job to be well informed about each resident, including name, age, physical and mental condition, daily medication, etc. By contrast, it seems that a large share of the residents do not even know the care workers' names. Another problem is that despite the great amount of occupational address terms in Japanese, no such term for care workers exists. This is perhaps a reflection of the fact that this profession does not have a long history in Japan. Added by the fact that pronominal address in non-intimate relationships is highly unusual, this lexical gap makes it all but impossible to directly address a care worker without knowing her or his name.

4.1.2   *Vocative vs. referential address*

While access to knowledge goes some way to account for the differences in address behaviour of residents and staff, it is certainly not the only reason. At this point, we should look more closely into the distinction between vocative and referential address in the data. An example of vocative usage from the speech of the care workers is LN-*san kao aratte* 'LN-san, wash your face' (#25'44), where the address term is not syntactically imbedded into the sentence but used as what Schegloff (1968: 1093) has referred to as a 'summons item'. This substantially differs from the type of address in a sentence like LN-*san mo o-toire ikimasu?* 'Is LN-*san* [= you] going to the toilet, too?' (#87'23), where LN-*san* does not have a summons function but happens to be the grammatical subject of the sentence (and where, as the translation shows, a pronoun would normally be the only option in English).

Table 4.4 Vocative vs. referential use of address terms, residents vs. staff

Type of usage	Staff to residents	Residents to staff	Example
Vocative	227 (90%)	3 (13%)	LN-*san kao aratte* (#25'44) 'LN-*san*, wash your face'
Referential	25 (10%)	21 (87%)	LN-*san mo o-toire ikimasu?* (#87'23) 'Is LN-*san* [= you] going to the toilet, too?'
	252 (100%)	24 (100%)	

Note: In 28 of the staff's vocatives, *san* is lengthened into *sa:n*.

In order to gain a better understanding as to which type of usage occurs in the data to what extent, all occurrences of an address term were categorised into either vocative or referential. In total, the 107 interactions contain 252 instances where a care worker addresses a resident. The large majority of these are used as vocatives, in a similar way as in the first example just presented. As can be seen in Table 4.4, 90% of the cases fall into this category. Conversely, an address term is used referentially in only 25 (10%) instances, as in the case of our second example.

This illustrates that address by the care workers predominantly functions as a call for a resident's attention. In line with this, it frequently occurs that the honorific suffix *san* is lengthened into a more call-like *sa:n*. No less than 28 instances (11%) in the speech of the care workers are marked by this feature, which appears to be particularly common in the opening of an interaction, as we will see in chapter 5 (see excerpts 5.1, 5.2, 5.3, 5.7).

A complementary look at the address terms used by the residents towards the care workers shows that the situation could not be more different here. As also shown in Table 4.4, the ratio for the two types of address is almost reversed in the case of the residents, who in the overall majority of the cases use terms of address in a referential way. Another noteworthy point is that the absolute numbers for referential address by both groups are conspicuously close, with 21 cases on the part of the residents and 25 cases on the part of the care workers, despite the fact that the care workers use more than ten times as many terms of address as the residents!

Taken together, this suggests that there is a small but sizable number of address terms used referentially to similar extent by both groups for 'grammatical' reasons. For instance, the referential use of the address term in the example presented above results from the structural necessity that the particle *mo* 'also, too' cannot stand on its own but has to be attached to a referent. The vast gap in the overall number of address terms, then, arises from the fact that the care workers mainly use them as vocatives, and that this way of summoning the interactional partner is not normally an option for the residents.

This relates to Weinhold's (1997) findings in a study on nurse–patient interaction in a German hospital. She observes that the quantitative differences in the use of nominal address (which in a German context factually means vocative address) between care workers and patients illustrate how the former are in charge, both of the workflow and of the talk (Weinhold 1997: 185). We will come back to this aspect of interactional control on various occasions throughout the analysis in the subsequent chapters.

4.1.3   Residents' address choices

The remainder of this section examines more closely those 24 rather exceptional cases where a resident does use a term of address, either referentially or, very rarely, as a vocative. All interactions that contain such instances are listed in Table 4.5, which shows that the most frequent address term is LN-*san* (#11, #84, #98, #99, #107), sometimes in combination with other forms such as *anta* (#59) or *otaku* (#26). Other options are pronouns only (#37, #97), the nominal honorific term *sensei* 'teacher, professor, doctor' (#46), and a (female) care worker's first name plus the hypercoristic person suffix -*chan*, in combination with the pronoun *omae* (#82). As becomes obvious here, although the residents rarely use terms of address at all, their choice is far more variegated than that of the care workers, who rely almost exclusively on first or last name address when they address the residents.

However, a closer look at Table 4.5 also reveals that almost half of the cases (#11, #46, #59, #82, #99) feature one specific speaker, Rm093. He is a man in his late 70s, who like most residents uses a wheelchair, but otherwise is still relatively independent. He is one of the first residents the care workers attend

Table 4.5 Address terms used by the residents (n=24)

Transcript number	Resident	Staff	Term(s) of address			
			Name	Pronoun	Other	
#11	Rm093	Sf4	LN-*san*			
#26	Rm094	Sf6	LN-*san* (2x)	*anta*	*otaku*	
#37	Rf053	Sf5		*anta*		(see excerpt 6.15)
#46	Rm093	Sm1			*sensei*	
#59	Rm093	Sm2	LN-*san* (7x)	*anta*		
#82	Rm093	Sf5	FN-*chan* (3x)	*omae*		(see excerpt 4.1)
#84	Rf162	Sf5	LN-*san*			
#97	Rf051	Sf3		*anata*		(see excerpt 5.15)
#98	Rf112	Sf3	LN-*san*			
#99	Rm093	Sm1	LN-*san*			
#107	Rf112	Sm1	LN-*san*			

to in the morning, and on their arrival they will already find him wide awake. Unlike many of the other residents, Rm093 shows a vivid and explicit interest in what is going on in Edogawa Care, including the people working and living there. The morning care activities seem to provide a welcome opportunity for him to learn about these matters from the staff.

Particularly noteworthy about Rm093's address behaviour is interaction #82, in which he calls the station nurse Sf5 three times by her first name. And instead of the standard person honorific -*san* suffix, he adds the -*chan* ending, which is most commonly used when talking to children. For adults, it is largely restricted to female addressees, usually to invoke some sort of smallness or cuteness. The passage in question is presented in excerpt 4.1.

It is just after 5:00 a.m. when the care worker enters the resident's room, opens the interaction with a greeting and asks him if he would like to get up. Excerpt 4.1 starts briefly after the opening phase, and in direct reaction to it. After being asked by the care worker why he is laughing, the resident in line 18 explains that he has been waiting for her for some time without using the nurse call. He refers to the care worker in this turn by the very informal pronoun *omae*, which already serves to invoke a rather intimate, non-institutional relationship between the two.

After the care worker's somewhat reserved acknowledgment and a standard token of apology (lines 19–20), both of which seem to have a distancing function, the resident in line 22 goes on to explain the reason for his refraining from using the nurse call: because FN-*chan* is 'such a poor girl' (which is as close as we get to the Japanese term *kawaisoo*, 'poor' for reasons other than money). The care worker on her part, laughingly but resolutely, rejects the resident's view of the situation by telling him that she is 'not a poor girl' at all (line 25).

Excerpt 4.1 (#82'18–25)

18	Res	*omae kuru made damattetan da yo=* I've kept silent until you came
19	CW	*=assoo:,* I see
20		*omachidoosama* Sorry for making you wait
21		(1.5, start of activities)
22	Res	*FN-chan kawaisoo dakara* [*yo* Because you're such a poor girl
23	CW	[*nande yo::* ((laughing)) What do you mean?
24		((laughs))
25		*kawaisoo ja nai yo* I'm not a poor girl

The resident's choice of the FN-*chan* address in this excerpt effectively contributes to foregrounding this 'poorness' of the care worker as he perceives it. His concern for the care worker, and the very explicit way he presents it to her, seems to temporarily reverse the interlocutors' roles as carer and cared-for: From the point of view of the resident, it is him who 'cares' for FN-*chan* rather than the other way round. The care worker's laughter, as her first reaction to this claim (lines 23–24), can be seen as a way of showing resistance to this view (Glenn 2003: 141–144).

This brings home one general point about terms of address frequently made in previous research in institutional settings: Language users do not blindly follow any predetermined rules of appropriateness in their choice of linguistic forms, but know how to bend and stretch these rules in order to express their local understanding of the special circumstances they find themselves in, and their relationship to the person that is in with them.

4.2 Speech level

Speech level is the most important component of Japanese addressee honorifics. Largely simplifying, one can make a basic distinction between a plain speech style that expresses intimacy and closeness, and a formal speech style for more distanced relationships. Grammatically, the difference between the two is indicated in verb endings and in the copula. Verbs in the formal style end in -*masu* or an inflected form thereof; the formal copula is *desu* and has similar inflections. That is why the formal style is also referred to as *desu/masu* style. Henceforth, I use the terms 'speech style' and 'speech level' interchangeably (see Usami 2015 for a discussion).

The formal style served as one of the earliest counter-examples to the universal claims of Brown and Levinson's (1987) concept of linguistic politeness. According to their framework, the main function of politeness is to abate the face threats inherent in social encounters. This can be done either by stressing intimacy and common ground with the other person, which is classified as positive politeness, or by showing concern for the other person's autonomy and freedom of action, which qualifies as negative politeness.

In a paper published in 1988, Matsumoto argued that the conceptualisation of politeness as a device to diminish face threats could not account for the use of the formal style in Japanese, as it is frequently required to mark sentences as formal even when they do not involve any face threats whatsoever. A similar point was made by Ide (1989), who distinguished between volition and 'discernment' and held that politeness in western cultures was mainly motivated by the former. By contrast, according to Ide, in Japanese and other eastern cultures, it is considered more important to 'discern' one's social position in a speech situation and behave accordingly (for a discussion, see Pizziconi 2003, 2011, Heinrich 2015).

Empirical research in both institutional and non-institutional settings has revealed that the use and non-use of the formal style is a highly complex problem that can be captured in its entirety neither by Brown and Levinson's politeness framework nor by Ide's concept of discernment. Settings that have been examined include casual conversations between friends (Maynard 1991, Itakura 2015), family interactions (Cook 1997), children's plays (Nakamura 2001, Fukuda 2005), neighbourhood quarrels (Cook 1999), first-encounter (Usami 2002, Tsuda 2010, Obana 2016) and multi-encounter conversations (Nakayama 2003), company meetings (Tanaka 2011), sales talk (Okamoto 1998), work place interactions (Saito 2010, 2011), interviews (David 2009), interactions in various academic and semi-academic settings (Okamoto 1997, 1999, Megumi 2002, Taniguchi 2004, Cook 2008, Geyer 2008a, 2008b, Hudson 2011, Enyo 2015), telephone conversations (Ishizaki 2000, Sugita 2004: 172–183, Obana 2016), computer mediated communication (Fukushima 2009, Miyake 2009, Nakamura 2009), TV talk shows and interviews (Ikuta 1983, Cook 1999, Tanaka 2004: 116–121), TV commercials (Murata 2004: 8–10), and prose and dialogues in fictional work (Maynard 1991, 2001: 18–28, Janes 2000, Barke 2010, 2011), among others.

Taken together, these studies have identified three basic functions of the two styles. First, and in line with most textbook explanations, choice between the formal and the plain style is based on the social relationship between the interlocutors, particularly in terms of status, gender, age, degree of intimacy, and overall formality of the situation. This closely corresponds to Ide's concept of 'discernment'. However, as such rather static constraints can hardly account for the pervasive phenomenon of intra-conversational style shifting, the marking of psychological distance has been identified as a second, more dynamic factor. According to this view, speech style can function as a device to assess and renegotiate the relationship between the interlocutors on a moment-by-moment basis. Third, researchers have explored the discursive functioning of the two styles in foregrounding and backgrounding certain types of information, expressing differing stances, epistemic modes and degrees of addressee awareness, and structuring the interactional flow.

In the care context, speech level has been examined by Furuta and Horie (2011, 2014). As described in section 2.3, they analysed 20 staff–resident interactions audio-recorded during the bathing routines in a Japanese eldercare facility. The authors identified the speech level for each utterance in the data and determined which one was predominantly used by the participants, with special focus on the speech of the care workers. They found that the plain style was clearly more prominent than the formal style, for which they suggest various reasons. One is that it is easier to give instructions in plain style, particularly when dealing with residents with a higher care level. In addition, the plain style may help reduce the psychological distance between care worker and care recipient. This is quantitatively supported by the fact that the plain style was particularly prominent during tasks of high intimacy, such as washing a resident's body. As for shifts to the formal style, Furuta and Horie (2014) discuss one situation of conflict where formal speech seems to be used to keep up the distance between the interactants. In addition, a shift to the formal style frequently occurred when an upcoming task was to be announced – an observation that testifies to the important discourse-organising function of speech style choices.

4.2.1 *Average rate of formal speech*

For the quantitative analysis of the present data, all occurrences of the formal style in the transcripts were coded. Apart from all clear cases of *desu* and *masu*, formal utterances were defined to include the hortative forms -*mashoo* and *deshoo* (which is not without problems – see, e.g., Hasegawa 2010: 144 note 4, Megumi 2002: 218), the request form V-*te kudasai*, and various formulaic expressions such as *ohayoo gozaimasu* 'Good morning', *arigatoo gozaimasu* 'Thank you', and *gomen nasai* 'I'm sorry'. Also counted as formal was the *ssu* form, an abbreviated version of copula *desu* to which we will come back below. Table 4.6 gives a list of the most common occurrences of the formal style according to this classification, juxtaposed to the forms that would qualify as their non-formal equivalents.

In order to calculate the percentage of utterances in formal style, the number of all lines marked as formal in a transcript was divided by that transcript's total number of lines. Excluded from the calculation were lines that did not contain transcribed speech (meta-comments, pauses, etc.) and lines from sequences in which the two main participants talked to someone else than each other.

No sub-classifications were made for non-formal speech, meaning that this category includes both utterances that are clearly marked for plain style and utterances that are not grammatically identifiable as plain, such as noun endings (*taigendome*) and other types of elliptic constructions. In addition, the non-formal category includes backchannel tokens, yes–no answers, one-word instructions, heave-hoes (see section 6.1.4), and other types of interjections for which

Table 4.6 Formal and non-formal utterances (model examples)

Classified as		Gloss
Formal	*Non-formal*	
moo sugu roku ji desu	*moo sugu roku ji (da yo)*	It's almost 6 o'clock.
okimasu	*okiru*	[I/we/you]'ll get up.
okimasen/okinai desu	*okinai*	[I/we/you] won't get up.
okimashoo	*okiyoo*	Let's get up.
okiru deshoo	*okiru daroo*	You're getting up, right?
okite kudasai	*okite*	(Please) get up.
ohayoo gozaimasu	*ohayoo*	Good morning.
arigatoo gozaimasu	*arigatoo*	Thank you.
gomen nasai	*gomen (ne)*	I'm sorry.
mooshiwake nai ssu	*mooshiwake nai*	I'm sorry.

Table 4.7 Average rate of formal speech

By	Average
Staff	12.3%
Residents	8.0%
All	**11.2%**

Table 4.8 Staff's average of formal speech

Care worker	Average
Sm1 (male)	2.3%
Sf6 (female)	8.7%
Sf4 (female)	12.1%
Sf3 (female)	12.1%
Sf5 (female)	18.6%
Sm2 (male)	26.5%

formal equivalents are hard to come up with. While this rather coarse-grained approach proved to be a workable solution to capture the overall degree of formality during the morning care routines, it needs to be kept in mind that only a small portion of what was classified as non-formal here is explicitly marked as plain in style.

Table 4.7 gives the average rate of formality in the speech of the residents and the staff in the 107 interactions. The fact that only 11.2% of the countable lines can be identified as formal means that, in reverse, almost 90% of what is said in the interactions is not delivered in *desu/masu* style. Even if only a part of these utterances grammatically qualifies as plain in style, this shows that a non-formal way of speaking is clearly the default mode between residents and staff during the morning care. To put this into context, a larger study of various (white-collar) work settings found that no less than 26.2% of all utterances were marked as formal style (Sasa 2002).

We now take a closer look at the average rate of formality for each of the six care workers, similarly calculated by dividing all of a care worker's transcript lines in formal style by the total number of lines transcribing her or his speech. As presented in Table 4.8, there are some huge individual differences. The care worker with the lowest formality average uses the formal style in only 2.3% of his utterances. By contrast, no less than 26.5% of the utterances by the care worker with the highest rate of formality are delivered in formal style. Remarkable about these two extremes is that both of them feature one of the two male care workers, Sm1 (lowest) and Sm2 (highest). In comparison, the averages of the four female care workers are much less divergent, with a range from 8.7% to 18.6% of lines in formal style.

These results show that the folk assumption that women tend to use more formal speech than men (e.g., Mizutani and Mizutani 1987, Ide and Yoshida 1999, but also see SturtzSreetharan 2006) does not hold for the present data. If there is a recognisable gender difference at all, it is that there is less variation in the degree of formality in the female care workers' speech than there is in the speech of their male colleagues. The next section will examine this variation in male speech in more detail.

4.2.2　Differences in male speech

The pronounced difference in the speech style of the two male care workers can best be understood if we compare two sequences of similar contents, presented in excerpts 4.2 and 4.3. In both cases, one of the care workers asks a female resident about the previous night, which – again in both cases – was rather restless, due to the resident's frequent visits to the toilet. Thus we have the same gender constellations, the same topic, and basically the same speech context.

Excerpt 4.2　(#102'8–20)

8	Res	[*un*
		((backchannel for earlier turn))
9	CW	*ne*[*e, sugoi toire ikisugi ja nai?*
		Haven't you been to the toilet far too much? ((plain))
10		(1.0)
11		*kyoo:,*
		Today
12	Res	°*un*°?
		What?
13		(0.5)
14	CW	*unn: nemureta no?*
		Uh-huh. Could you sleep? ((plain))
15	Res	*nemui*
		I'm sleepy. ((plain))
16	CW	*e?*
		What?
17	Res	*nemui*
		I'm sleepy. ((plain))
18	CW	*nemui? nemureta?*
		You're sleeply? ((plain)) Could you sleep? ((plain))
19		(0.5)
20		*nemureta no ne*
		So you could sleep then. ((plain))

Excerpt 4.3 (#60'19–33)

19	CW	*kinoo neremashita:?*
		Could you sleep yesterday? ((formal))
20		(1.0)
21	Res	°*nemuremasen deshita ne*°
		I couldn't sleep ((formal))
22	CW	*nemasen deshita ne:* (0.8)
		You didn't sleep, did you? ((formal))
23		*soo desu yo ne*
		That's right, isn't it? ((formal))
24		(1.2)
25		*daitai/ dde are desu yo,*
		Mostly you were like, ((formal))
26		*ano: kinoo wa* (1.0)
		well yesterday was
27		*e:to ne:,* (1.6)
		well,
28		*yoru hachi ji kurai kara:,* (0.8)
		from about eight in the evening,
29		*ni jikan oki ni,*
		every two hours
30		*toire deshita kara ne*
		it was toilet ((formal))
31	Res	*a:*
		Uh:
32	CW	*a:.* ((laughs))
		Uh:.
33		*sonna ni nete nai ja nai ssu ka ne*
		You didn't sleep that much, did you? ((formal))

Excerpt 4.2 gives the sequence with Sm1, the care worker with the lowest average of formal speech. Note that the excerpt does not contain a single utterance in the formal style. Conversely, a large portion of the care worker's utterances is unambiguously marked as plain (lines 9, 14, 18, and 20). This is in stark contrast to the sequence in excerpt 4.3, which features the other male care worker. In this excerpt, virtually all of the syntactically complete turns are marked as formal (lines 19, 22, 23, 25, 30, 33). Of further note is that in both cases, the residents seem to adapt to the speech style chosen by the staff. The resident in excerpt 4.2 uses the plain style to reply to the care worker's plain question if she could properly sleep (lines 15 and 17). By contrast, the resident in excerpt 4.3 when asked about the same issue in the formal style delivers her reply in the formal style, too (line 21).

What the two sequences further have in common is that the speech of the care workers in both cases contains an element of reproach regarding the resident's high number of toilet visits and, implicitly, the additional work this caused during the night. However, as can be understood from the two transcripts, the reproach comes across in a much more careful and less face-threatening way in excerpt 4.3. To be sure, this is not merely a result of the care worker's use of the formal style. Other factors include a more neutral opening question (line 19), the use of hesitation markers (lines 25, 26, 27), approximators (lines 25, 28), and hedges (line 33), as well as the care worker's somewhat awkward laughter (line 32). However, his choice of the formal speech style takes a chief part in playing down the overall force of the reproach.

Another noteworthy point in the speech of Sm2 is his shortening of the formal copula *desu* into *ssu* in line 33. This so-called 'novel honorific' (*shinkeigo*), a phenomenon documentable since the 1960s (Kuramochi 2009: 26), is a comparatively common feature in his speech. The sample contains a total of 26 instances of the form, no less than 19 of which occur in utterances by Sm2. As previous studies have shown, the main function of the *ssu* form is to reduce the in-built distancing of the formal speech style without having to fall back on the directness of plain speech (e.g., Kuramochi 2009, Nagatomi 2012). This may be the most likely reason why Sm2 tends to intersperse his speech with forms like *mada makkura ja nai ssu ka* 'It's still pitch dark, isn't it?' (#59'165), *ase sugoi ssu ne* 'That's a lot of sweat' (#61'55), or, as in excerpt 4.3, *sonna ni nete nai ja nai ssu ka ne* 'You didn't sleep that much, did you?'

4.2.3 Speech level shifts

The quantitative analysis and the two excerpts just discussed serve to demonstrate that there are some rather pronounced individual differences in the usage and non-usage of addressee honorifics. However, this does not capture the more 'messy reality' (Jones and Ono 2008) of shifts between the two styles. As mentioned in the introductory part of this section, such shifts are highly common in Japanese interaction, and the present data are by no means an exception. While it is unrealistic to take hold of the phenomenon in its entirety here, excerpt 4.4 presents one longer sequence that exemplifies how both the care workers and the residents use style shifts to indicate differing stances and interactional modalities as they are working their way through the morning care tasks.

The excerpt starts while the care worker is wheeling the resident from his room to the toilet. As they are moving along, the care worker coughs several times. This is commented on by the resident in line 62, noting that all of the 'young people' seem to be having a cold. After a confirmative reply by the care worker (line 63), and partially in overlap with it, the resident starts explaining why he thinks this might be the case: because of the staff's irregular sleeping times (lines 64–65). He is referring here to the short break in the nap room that each of the two care workers takes at some point during the night. At least, that is how the care worker interprets his statement, as becomes clear in the subsequent part of the sequence.

Excerpt 4.4 (#40'61–84)

61	CW	(9.0, to toilet, coughs several times)
62	Res	*wakai hito mina-san kaze hiiteru no ne* The young people are all having a cold, don't they
63	CW	*nandaka ne, kyuu ni* [*ne:::* somehow, right, all of a sudden,
64	Res	[*okitari okitari okitari=* Getting up getting up getting up
65		=*netari okitari netari* sleeping, getting up, sleeping
66	CW	((laughs))
67		*watashi-tachi sokon/,* We don/
68		*sonna ni takusan nete nai desu yo* don't sleep that much there actually. ((formal))
69	Res	*unn* Uh-huh
70	CW	*samukattari* [*ne, atatakattari ga ne,* It's cold and then it's warm again, you see
71	Res	[*a:sososoo:* Oh yeah
72	CW	*kurikaeshite ne*[: over and over again
73	Res	[*soo deshoo* Yeah, that must be it.
74		(2.5)
75		*soriya taihen da yo ne* That's really awful, isn't it?
76		(0.6)
77	CW	*ne:::* Isn't it?
78		(4.5)
79		*baka wa kaze hikanai tte iu no ni ne=* Though they say idiots don't catch a cold
80		=*kaze hiichatta yo* I did just that
81		(1.2)
82		*hai, doozo* Okay, here you go
83	Res	*sonna koto nai desu* [*yo* No, that's not true. ((formal))
84	CW	[((laughs))

Up to here, the whole passage has been in non-formal style. The shift occurs in line 68, when the care worker after a false start in the previous line finds it necessary to clarify that we 'don't sleep that much' during the shift. Her use of the formal style cuts off this utterance from the rest of the ongoing talk, as though to grammatically distance herself from what the resident has just said. Further adding to this effect is the pluralised first person pronoun *watashi-tachi* 'we' in her turn in line 67. Used non-inclusively here, it draws a line between the group of the care workers or, in the words of the resident, 'the young people' (line 62) and the care recipients. This has a similarly distancing function as her shift to the formal style. Note that the passage in question is preceded by the care worker's laughter (line 66), which serves to both prepare and soften her upcoming disagreement.

After an acknowledgment by the resident (line 69), the care worker continues by providing a different reason for why she and her colleagues tend to get sick around this time of year: It is because of the temperature differences they are faced with during work (line 70, also see excerpt 6.15). Having once expressed her disagreement rather explicitly, she now seems to be going out of her way to deemphasise the differences with the resident's point of view and re-establish common ground. She does so by recycling much of the grammatical and semantic material from his previous turn in lines 64 and 65: the *-tari* construction, which is used for non-exhaustive listings of actions or states, as well as the juxtaposing of the antonyms 'warm' and 'cold', which mimics the resident's 'getting up' and 'sleeping'. In addition, and most relevant for the present discussion, she shifts back to a non-formal way of speaking to show that she is 'back with him'.

The resident expresses his agreement with her view through backchannelling (lines 71 and 73) and a summarising assessment that this must be 'awful' (line 75). A token of acknowledgment by the care worker in line 77 concludes the sequence. This leads to a pause of 4.5 seconds, after which the care worker initiates a follow-up on the topic: that despite the common Japanese saying that 'idiots don't catch a cold', she did just that (lines 79–80). This is a negative self-assessment that would call for a quick disagreement by the conversational partner (Pomerantz 1984a). And although it takes a pause of 1.2 seconds and another task-related turn by the care worker (lines 81–82), the resident finally does reject the care worker's self-assessment (line 83). He chooses the formal style to do so, again in contrast to the preceding part of the sequence. Here, too, the temporary resort to the formal style can be seen as a device that sets the utterance apart from the previous stage of the conversation, including the care worker's negative self-assessment, in order to express the required disagreement with what has just been said.

As the sequence in excerpt 4.4 illustrates, occasional shifts from non-formal to formal speech fulfil an important function in fine-tuning and recalibrating the relationship between the participants as the interaction unfolds. In line with most recent studies on Japanese addressee honorifics, this shows that speakers in interactions take advantage of this honorific device to express their understanding of the situation on a turn-by-turn basis, rather than adhering to any wholesale rules about formal and informal speech and their relative position vis-à-vis the other person.

4.3 Referent honorifics

A third important component of Japanese politeness grammar is referent honorifics. They differ from speech level choice, at least in theory, as they do not mark the relationship with the person spoken to, but refer to the person that is spoken about. Although these two vanishing points frequently coincide (because addressee and referent more often than not are the same person), the two types of honorifics can be conceptualised independent of each other. An overall distinction can be made between forms used to exalt others and forms that function to humble oneself or one's in-group. In addition, there is a specific morphological device used for linguistic beautification, which is located at the borderline between referent and addressee honorifics.

This section examines the occurrence of all three types of honorifics in the data. Humilifics and exalting forms are explored in section 4.3.1, followed by a closer look at the phenomenon of beautification in section 4.3.2. We conclude by taking a look at the occurrence of the hyper-formal copula verb *gozaru* and the specific interactional effect it achieves, which is presented in section 4.3.3.

4.3.1 *Humilifics and exalting forms*

Both humble and exalting forms are marked mainly on verbs, in addition to a restricted number of nouns and adjectives. Forms to humble oneself or one's in-group include different lexemes, if available, and periphrastic constructions based on the prefixes *o* or *go* and the verb *suru* 'do'. A sub-distinction can be made depending on whether a humbling expression signalises the speaker's relationship to the referent or that to the addressee (Bunkacho 2007), which shows that this type of honorific has some qualities of addressee honorifics as well (also see Traugott and Dasher 2002: 258–263, Matsumoto 2014).

For forms that exalt the other person or that person's in-group, a number of separate lexemes are available, too. In addition, virtually every verb can be used in the passive voice to express an exalting attitude towards others' actions. As with humble forms, there is also a periphrastic construction, again using the prefixes *o* and *go* but with the verb *naru* 'become'. Accessible overviews on the topic are provided in Niyekawa (1991: chapter 4), Tranter and Kizu (2012: 301–302), Iwasaki (2013: 320–325), and Hasegawa (2015: 258–267).

In the present data, both humble and exalting forms are relatively scarce. The most frequent humilific constructions are highly lexicalised phrases like *o-negai shimasu* 'please', sometimes upgraded to *o-negai itashimasu*, and *o-matase shimashita*, which is a standard phrase to acknowledge having kept someone waiting. It can be found in the data a total of eight times and is used only by the care workers, reflecting the obvious fact that it is normally them, not the residents, who 'make wait'.

A third humilific in the data is the apology formula *shitsurei itashimasu*, which in past tense becomes *shitsurei itashimashita* or, in one case, *shitsurei itashiyashita*. This last form deserves some special attention with respect to the interplay between referent and addressee honorifics. According to Nakamura (2007: 71–72), the phonemic shift from V-*masu* to V-*yasu* (and, in past tense, V-*mashita* to V-*yashita*) is motivated by the same process that in adjectives and noun constructions turns the formal copula *desu* into the 'novel honorific' *ssu* (see section 4.2.2). The form *shitsurei itashiyashita*, then, is basically a combination of a humilific referent honorific and a not entirely formal (and not entirely serious) addressee honorific, resulting in an intentional 'mismatch' of the two levels. We will come back to a similar construction in the course of the discussion.

The sample also contains a small number of humilific expressions based on the benefactive verb *itadaku* (as opposed to its neutral correspondent *morau* 'receive'). It serves to express a humble acknowledgment that something is being done for oneself (V-*te itadaku*) or that one's action is implicitly contingent on the other's approval (V-*(s)asete itadaku*) (Shioda 2016: 32–39, Onoda 2016d: 164). This type of humilific is used exclusively by the residents.

As the examples here presented show, humilific forms predominantly occur in routinised speech acts involving an apology or similar acknowledgment of causing an imposition on the other person. Excerpt 4.5 presents one longer sequence

Excerpt 4.5 (#97'1–13)

1	CW	((enters room))
2		LN-*san ohayoo gozaima*[:*su*
		LN-san, Good morning
3	Res	[*ohayoo go*/=
		Good mor/
4		=*yoroshiku onegai itashimasu*
		((in-advance gratitude formula)) ((humble))
5		*suimasen de (goza*/) (0.6)
		((apology formula, aborted))
6		*go-meiwaku o okake* [*itashimashite*
		((apology for inconveniences)) ((humble))
7	CW	[(((clearing her throat))
8		(0.6)
9	Res	[°##°
10	CW	[*o-toire ikaremasu*?
		Are you going to the toilet? ((exalting))
11	Res	*ee, chotto o-toire yo*/
		Yes, I'd just
12		[*yorasete itadakimasu*
		like to do drop by there a little ((humble))
13	CW	[*ha:i*
		Okay

that exemplifies how this is done in interaction. It features a female resident who makes comparatively heavy use of humilific forms in all four of the interactions she is involved in.

The excerpt gives the first few moments of the exchange, starting with the care worker entering the resident's room. After the care worker's opening greeting has been reciprocated by the resident (lines 2–3), there follows a whole battery of quickly delivered (and in part unfinished) standard phrases that foreground the resident's awareness of the inconveniences she is causing to the care worker. Of these, the phrases *yoroshiku o-negai itashimasu* and *go-meiwaku o o-kake itashimashite* in lines 4 and 6 contain humilifics. Morphologically speaking, each of the two is marked as humble twice, since both are based on the humilific construction *o* V-*suru* but additionally replace *suru* by its humilific correspondent *itasu*. A third humble form is used by the resident in line 12, in reaction to the care worker's question if she would like to go to the toilet. Her affirmative reply combines the causative form of the verb *yoru* 'drop by' with the humilific benefactive *itadaku*.

However, the resident does not solely rely on referent honorifics to express her indebtedness to the care worker. In addition, she consistently uses the formal style and delivers her speech in a low, almost whispering voice, as though to make herself not only grammatically but also acoustically smaller. Another point with respect to prosody is that she speaks very quickly, thus showing an awareness that she does not want to take up more of the care worker's time than necessary. This may also be the main reason for why she aborts her greeting halfway through and moves right on to express her in-advance gratitude (lines 3–4). Of further note is her use of the verb *yoru* 'drop by' rather than *iku* 'go', in combination with the adverb *chotto* 'a little' (line 11–12), which can be seen as an attempt to verbally downsize the care worker's burden of taking her to the toilet (Matsumoto 1985, 2001). Taken together, it becomes obvious here how the resident goes out of her way to communicate to the care worker that she is aware of the inconveniences she causes, and will do her utmost to keep them to a minimum. Humilific forms are but one of a number of devices to express this, but they are an important one.

One remarkable point in the sequence is that the resident's excessive use of referent honorifics seems to have some spillover effect on the speech of the care worker, who hardly ever uses such forms elsewhere in the data. The present interaction is rather exceptional in that she formulates her question about going to the toilet by using the exalting passive *ikareru* (rather than *iku* 'go'), which in formal style becomes *ikaremasu* (line 10). This is another instance where we can observe how the honorific levels of the two participants' speech seem to converge.

Continuing with exalting honorifics, one basic thing to note is that, as in the example just discussed, such forms occur almost exclusively in the speech of the care workers. They are most often used for making a request (though, as we will see in chapter 6, they are not the standard format for this type of speech act). Examples are *o-tachi kudasai* 'Please stand up', *o-kake kudasai* 'Please sit down' (also see excerpt 6.6), and *o-machi kudasai* 'Please wait'. This last one is particularly common when a care worker answers an incoming nurse call. Of all 15 cases where the phrase occurs, 11 are made in reply to a resident calling from another room and thus not directed at the physically present participant. To some extent at least, the frequent use of the humble form here may result from the 'telephonic' nature of the exchange, which seems to call for a stylistically more refined register than the concurrent face-to-face interaction.

A second context where exalting honorifics can occur is when topics related to the residents are discussed. In one example, given in excerpt 4.6, a care

Excerpt 4.6 (#83'37–55)

37	CW	*demo sono ato o-uchi chokotto=*
		But after that you're
38		*=yotte kurun [deshoo*
		dropping in at your place, right? ((exalting))
39	Res	[*soo desu ne:=*
		Yes, that's right
40	CW	*=unn*
		Uh-huh
41		(1.1)
42	Res	*kaeri wa hiru kara ni narimasu*
		I won't be back over the day
43	CW	*a:soo desu ka*
		I see.
44		(1.0)
45		*yuushoku tabete kaette=*
		Have dinner outside and
46	Res	*=soo de[su ne=*
		Right
47	CW	[(*#ne*),
		Right
48	Res	*hai=*
		Yes
49	CW	*=un*
		Uh-huh
50		(0.9)
51		*ii mono tabete kite kudasai yo*
		Be sure you have something good to eat
52		(1.7)
53		*musuko-san ja kyoo wa o-yasumi=*
		So your son has taken
54		*=totte kuda[satta no?*
		a day off then? ((exalting))
55	Res	[*unn, soo desu ne*
		Uh-huh, that's right

worker and a resident are talking about the resident's plans for the day. As the care worker knows, he is going to have an outpatient check-up at a nearby hospital in the morning, to which his son will accompany him. After that, as we learn in the excerpt, they will drop by at the son's (and the resident's former) place, and in the evening have dinner together.

In this sequence, the care worker chooses the exalting forms *o-uchi* 'your place' (line 37) and *o-yasumi totte kudasatta* '(your son) took a day off (for you)' (lines 53–54). Interesting about the second expression is that, in contrast to most of the other utterances in this sequence, she uses it in plain style (*kudasatta* rather than *kudasaimashita*). The result is an honorific hybrid that combines an exalting reference form with the non-formal speech style. As has been noted in previous studies, such hybrids are commonly ascribed to female speakers. They serve to fine-tune the balance between expressing respect and intimacy (e.g., Ide and Yoshida 1999: 478, Hasegawa 2010: 142), in a way similar to the previously described V-*yasu* form. We will come back to these instances of honorific blending in the discussion at the end of the chapter.

4.3.2 Beautification

The last component of Japanese honorifics to be discussed here is beautification expressions. Adding *o* or *go* prefixes before nouns and adjectives, these constructions are formally indistinguishable from exalting forms like the just mentioned *o-uchi* or *o-yasumi*. However, they are not confined to talk about the other person's sphere, but can be used for the sole purpose of expressing a formal speech attitude as such. That is why, strictly speaking, beautification expressions qualify as addressee rather than referent honorifics. They have been included in this section on account of their morphological similarity with exalting expressions, in addition to the fact that the distinction between 'mere' stylistic beautification and referent beautification is anything but straightforward.

Beautification expressions in the data include terms such as *o-kusuri* 'medicine', *o-futon* 'blanket', *o-mizu* 'water', and *o-furo* 'bath'. In addition, the data contain a large number of taboo expressions that commonly take the shape of beautified forms, including *o-tearai* 'toilet', *o-shiri* 'a person's back', *o-naka* 'stomach' and *o-shikko* 'pee'. Some of these have become lexicalised to an extent that the beautification prefix is virtually obligatory.

By far the most common beautification expression is *o-toire* 'toilet', which occurs in the data a total of 53 times. In contrast to many other taboo expressions, the beautification prefix is not obligatory here, perhaps owing to the loanword background of the term. The data contain no less than 92 cases of the 'plain', non-beautified form *toire*. A closer look at these two variants shows that there is a relatively pronounced gender bias. As can be seen in Table 4.9, female speakers, both residents and staff, use the two forms to almost equal extents. By contrast, the male speakers of the sample hardly ever add a beautification marker when they use the term. In total, there are only three instances of *o-toire* in male speech. Unlike with speech style, gender seems to be a recognisable factor here.

Table 4.9 Beautified and non-beautified uses of the term *toire* 'toilet'

	o-toire (beautified)		toire (non-beautified)		Total	
Females	50	51.5%	47	48.5%	97	100.0%
Males	3	6.3%	45	93.8%	48	100.0%
Sum	**53**	**36.6%**	**92**	**63.4%**	**145**	**100.0%**

Excerpt 4.7 (#47'31–34)

31	CW	*hai o-toire* [*iku yo*
		Okay we're going to the toilet ((beautified))
32	Res	[##
33		(1.8)
34	CW	*toire iku yo*
		We're going to the toilet ((non-beautified))

Regarding the three male *o-toire* cases, it may be somewhat surprising that all of them are produced by Sm1, the care worker who makes least frequent use of the formal style (see section 4.2). One example is presented in excerpt 4.7, where Sm1 announces to a female resident he has just helped out of bed that he will now take her to the toilet. Noteworthy about his choice of *o-toire* in line 31 is that he uses it in combination with the plain style (*iku* rather than *ikimasu*). This mixture shows that the two types of addressee honorifics clearly lead a life independent of each other.

A second point of note is that when the care worker repeats his announcement in line 34, after a non-reconstructable reply by the resident, he uses the non-beautified form *toire*. The occurrence of both variants within the same sequence, by the same speaker and in close proximity of each other, suggests that the use of beautification devices cannot be properly appreciated if only extra-linguistic variables are taken into account. Rather, and in a similar way to speech style shifts, beautification seems to have some important, and as yet not entirely understood, interactional functions. In the present example, for instance, the stylistic downgrade when repeating the announcement about going to the toilet might be indicative of some sort of impatience on the part of the care worker. This is a point to be more closely examined when discussing tempo differences between residents and staff in section 7.3.

4.3.3 Honorific role language

One final aspect of honorifics that should not go unnoticed is their usage for the sake of humour and verbal play. An example is presented in excerpt 4.8, which starts with the opening greeting by a care worker who has just returned

Excerpt 4.8 (#89'1–23)

1	CW	((back after having accompanied other resident from this room to toilet))
2		*ohayoo gozansu* Good morning ((archaic))
3		(1.8)
4		*bochibochi rokuji de gozaru kedo* It's almost 6 o'clock ((archaic))
5		(0.8)
6	Res	°(##*ka*)°
7		(0.4)
8	CW	*hai?* What?
9		(0.5)
10	Res	*hai* Okay
11	CW	*bochibochi rokuji de gojaru* It's almost 6 o'clock ((archaic))
12	Res	*rokuji de gojaru* 6 o'clock ((archaic))
13	CW	((laughs)[)
14	Res	[((laughs))
15	CW	*doo nasaru ka* What are you going to do? ((archaic))
16		(0.9)
17	Res	*okiyansh[oo ka* Shall we get up then? ((archaic))
18	CW	[*okiyanshoo ka ne* Shall we get up then, right? ((archaic))
19	Res	(########)
20	CW	*kyoo wa Edokko-fuu ja nai?* Today we're in an old-style Tokyo mood, aren't we?
21		(0.5)
22		((laughs[))
23	Res	[((laughs))

from taking another resident from this room to the toilet. After her greeting on re-entry, she informs the resident that it is now almost 6 o'clock (line 4). From this develops an exchange oriented to reaching a mutual agreement about getting the resident out of bed. By the time the resident gives her explicit consent to the suggested course of action in line 17, this has largely been achieved.

A closer analysis of the structural features of openings in the data will be provided in the next chapter. Relevant for the present discussion is the occurrence of a couple of somewhat quaint honorific expressions involving the honorific copula verb *gozaru* and several of its variants: *gozansu* (instead of *gozaimasu*, line 2), *de gozaru* (instead of *desu* or *de gozaimasu*, line 4), and *de gojaru*, a further modified form of *de gozaru* (lines 11 and 12).

Whereas the copula *de gozaimasu* in hyper-formal speech is still in use in present-day Japanese, its non-formal correspondent *de gozaru* as it occurs in excerpt 4.8 is clearly a relic of the past (e.g., Twine 1991: 70–73, Uehara 2011: 206). Maynard (2004: 406) has referred to it as an 'imagined style', while Yamaguchi (1999: 40) calls it '*ninja* register' (see also Akizuki 2015). The form *nasaru ka* (line 15), which combines the exalting variant of *suru* 'do' with a rather unusual question format in plain style can be considered part of this register, too.

That the participants are fully aware of the 'off-ness' of their speech can be understood from the care worker's meta-comment that today they are 'in an old-style Tokyo mood' (line 20). Moreover, as their recurring laughter suggests (lines 13–14, 22–23), they seem to be quite enjoying this playing around with honorific 'role language' (Kinsui 2003, 2007) and the resulting mismatch with the quotidian content matter of their talk. Rather than expressing a higher degree of mutual respect, the use of honorifics here serves to create some humorous effect that helps deal with the interactionally precarious issue of compliance gaining (see section 5.1) and makes the interaction go smoothly. Though similar cases are rare in the data, they show that honorifics do much more than just express respect, formality, or a 'polite' attitude.

4.4 Discussion

This first part of the analysis has explored the data with respect to the occurrence of honorifics. Examining terms of address, we have started with a look at how the care workers commonly call the residents when they talk to them. A quantitative analysis has shown that the majority of the residents are consistently addressed by their last name plus the person honorific -*san*, which can be considered the default mode in the setting under observation. In addition, address by first name plus *san* is an option for a small group of – mainly female – residents. Gender seems to be a notable extralinguistic variable here.

When presenting these findings to the care workers in Edogawa Care at one of the study sessions, an additional factor they suggested for favouring first name address was 'ease of calling' (*yobiyasusa*). As one participant explained, particularly female residents whose first name had only two syllables and did not have the common *ko* (literally, 'child') ending might be likely candidates for first name address. When reviewing the data later on, it turned out that four of the six residents in question had such names. While a much larger data set would be required to generalise these findings, this suggests that intralinguistic factors may play their part in determining address choice, too.

Making a basic distinction between vocative and referential usage, the analysis has further revealed that the care workers use address terms mainly as vocatives. This suggests that terms of address fulfil an important function as call-outs to summon a resident's attention. The prominence of vocatives in the care workers' speech, often with the person suffix *san* lengthened into *sa:n*, can be seen as a manifestation of how they try to get – and maintain – hold of the interactional flow. In this respect, Blum-Kulka et al. (1989: 277) have found that terms of address frequently function as 'attention getters' in making requests. This being the case, it is perhaps worth noting that previous researchers have observed a functional similarity between vocatives and imperatives (Jakobson 1971: 10, Leech 1999: 109).

A last finding with respect to the care workers is that the fictive use of kinship terms is clearly not common practice in Edogawa Care. The data include only one case where a resident, in a situation of considerable emotional turmoil, is called *okaa-san* 'mother'. In addition, the non-transcribed parts of the data contain a few instances where a resident is jokingly addressed as *ojoo-san* 'daughter'. In general though, we can say that the fictive use of kinship terms is rare in the observed care setting, and that kinship terms indicative of old age do not occur at all. This is largely in line with my personal impression during the field observations in advance of and during the recordings. We should avoid generalisations though, as there seem to be care facilities where the fictive use of kinship terms is still quite common (see the examples presented in Kitamoto 2006, 2007).

The chief finding with respect to the residents' use of address terms is the comparative scarcity of such forms. Quantitatively speaking, only slightly more than 10% of all interactions contain a term of address towards a care worker. A similar imbalance applies to vocative vs. referential usage. In contrast to the care workers, the residents use terms of address mainly referentially. Recall that both groups produce almost the same absolute numbers of referential address terms. Seen in this light, the huge quantitative differences in address term usage seem to expose more profound differences as to who is in charge, and who is not. In this sense, vocative address is arguably one of the most obvious reflections of institutional power differences in the data.

Despite the low frequency of address terms by the residents, there is much greater variety in their speech than we find in the speech of the care workers. In part at least, this may be a result of the residents' not knowing a care worker's name, but it is clearly not the only factor. Of special note is the use of a number of rather intimate terms such as the very impersonal second person pronouns *omae* and *anta*, as well as the hypercoristic FN-*chan*. The example presented in excerpt 4.1 has shown how terms of address may be a useful device to break up the institutionally prescribed roles of the participants, at least temporarily, and redefine their relationship in different, more personal terms.

Moving on to speech style, a necessarily coarse-grained quantification has shown that a non-formal way of speaking is the default mode during the morning care activities in Edogawa Care. On the other hand, a closer look at the care workers' speech suggests that there are some pronounced individual differences. Of particular note are the two male care workers, who account for both the highest (Sm2) and the lowest (Sm1) ratio of formal speech. A comparison of two excerpts of similar content has demonstrated how the use and non-use of addressee honorifics – among a myriad of other devices – translates into considerably different interactional styles. We will come back to these intra-gender differences in the concluding chapter.

Any account of speech style would be incomplete without paying attention to the ubiquitous phenomenon of back-and-forth shifts between plain and formal speech. While it is beyond the scope of this study to capture the whole complexity of this phenomenon, the example presented in excerpt 4.4 has been intended to provide at least a glimpse of the different functions that style shifts may fulfil. Far from simply communicating different degrees of formality or other external conditions such as role or gender, we have seen that the two speech styles are used by the participants to organise the interaction and their temporary understanding of it 'on the spot'. As the subsequent chapters will further demonstrate, this 'discourse-organisational' function of style shifts (Maynard 1991) is of vital importance in talking while working, and working while talking.

Perhaps the most important finding with respect to referent honorifics in the data is that there is in fact not much to be found. As the analysis has shown, particularly humilific forms are largely confined to formulaic expressions such as *o-negai shimasu* or *o-matase shimashita* and hardly ever 'assembled' online. Exalting forms are used in a slightly more productive way, as the example discussed in excerpt 4.6 has demonstrated, but such cases are more an exception than the rule. Generally speaking, it is safe to say that neither humilific nor exalting forms are part of the common speech repertory in Edogawa Care.

The low frequency of referent honorifics concurs with the overall preference of non-formal over formal speech, suggesting that the default way of speaking in Edogawa Care is considerably casual in nature. On first look, this may be somewhat counter-intuitive, given the fact that the participants are adult speakers who in most cases have known each other for less than a few months, if not weeks. However, and corresponding with observations from previous research (e.g., Ōtani 2004: 88, Watanabe 2008: 183, Onoda 2016a: 86), it seems that the very intimate tasks to be performed by the participants in this setting call for a mode of speech that is much closer to family interaction than to the language of more prototypical service encounters. Conversely, it may well be that a more comprehensive use of honorifics would be all but incompatible with the intimacy of the care tasks. Simply put, you just do not exchange honorifics with people with whom you go to the toilet.

A few other parallels between addressee and referent honorifics are noticeable, too. One is larger individual differences. These manifest themselves not only in the drastically different speech styles of Sm1 and Sm2, as noted, but can also be found in the heavy usage of humbling forms by the resident featured in excerpt 4.5, which is quite exceptional in the data. Such outlier cases deserve special attention as they caution us against over-generalisations with respect to the uses and users of honorifics in Edogawa Care. On the other hand, the examples discussed also include various cases where the use of honorifics by two interlocutors seems to converge as they continue talking (excerpts 4.2, 4.3, 4.5, 4.8). This finding is in line with accommodation theory (e.g., Giles et al. 1991, Giles 2016), and quantitatively supported by the remarkably close averages of formal speech, with 12% for the care workers' utterances and 8% for the residents'.

A final correspondence between the two honorific levels is the way in which they may become blended and combined. Examples include the semi-formal *ssu* copula, humilific verbs ending in *-yashita* instead of *-mashita*, exalting forms that come in plain style, and the use of outdated forms for the sake of what I have referred to as honorific role language. As these instances show, the participants take advantage of the whole palette of available honorific colours to concoct what they deem the right 'tone' for each interactional moment. This goes far beyond any textbook ideas of demeanour and contextual appropriateness.

Taken together, the analysis of terms of address, speech style, and referent honorifics in this chapter demonstrates that there are a handful of external variables that seem to influence the occurrence of honorifics in Edogawa Care, in a classical, variationist sociolinguistic sense. With respect to institutional role, for instance, we have seen that vocative address is a prerogative of the care workers. Similarly, the analysis shows that a small number of residents make use of a greater variety of terms. Another factor to be considered is gender, which seems to account for the occurrence of first name address for residents. In addition, there is the clearly gender-distinct usage of beautification forms.

Yet on the other hand, the data reveal that there is great flexibility and creativity in the usage of honorifics, defying any oversimplified correlations between speakers' background variables and their linguistic output. The most straightforward example is addressee honorifics, use of which can be accounted for neither by gender nor by status or power. In this respect, one can only agree with Barke's (2010: 473, emphasis original) assessment that 'the *rules* for honorific usage are not determined by the *rules* for assessing external contextual factors. Rather, they tend to emerge from the repeated interactions and negotiations between interactants in their everyday activities'.

5 Openings and closings

Virtually all types of social encounters fall into three distinguishable parts: an opening phase that assures a coordinated entry into the interaction, a closing phase through which the participants make their exchange come to a mutually agreed ending, and a main part, sandwiched in between, which usually makes up the largest portion of the transaction. Based on this rather straightforward structure, the present chapter takes a closer look at the first two of the described components. Section 5.1 presents the basic organisation of the openings to morning care interaction in Edogawa Care and how they work to get things started. Section 5.2 explores the main properties of how the participants at the end of an exchange manage to take leave of each other in a coordinated way. An analysis of the middle part, which is chiefly oriented to the performance of the care tasks, will be provided in chapter 6.

5.1 Openings

Openings can be understood as 'solutions to the problem of how to begin an encounter' (Robinson 2013: 261). Trivial as it may seem, this involves a large number of organisational issues that need to be addressed before an interaction can proceed to the main part. Moreover, previous research has shown that the way an interaction is started may significantly pre-structure the way it unfolds.

An early study about the sequential organisation of openings is Schegloff's classic from 1968. Analysing audio-recordings of emergency calls to the police, Schegloff identified a basic summons–answer structure, which he found determined much of the subsequent development of the turn-taking. This mutually dependent call-and-response dyad later came to be referred to as one type of adjacency pair. Adjacency pairs minimally consist of an utterance (or other communicative action) by a first speaker, commonly referred to as first pair part (FPP), which requires some sort of reaction by a second speaker in the form of what is called a second pair part (SPP). Talk in interactions is largely structured by a constant recurrence of this pattern.

Schegloff observed that an interaction usually starts with some sort of 'attention-getting device'. This may be a term of address, a 'courtesy phrase' (e.g., 'Pardon me'), or some non-verbal action like waves of a hand or a tap on the shoulder.

In the case of telephone calls, the ringing of the phone fulfils this function. It constitutes the first pair part of an interaction's earliest possible adjacency pair. This makes a reaction by the receiver of the call a relevant next action, normally by answering the phone and thus providing the second pair part to the summons–answer sequence. The same mechanism also accounts for the basic rule that it is usually the person that answers the phone who speaks first (Schegloff 1968).

The characteristics of openings in institutional eldercare have been examined by Grainger (1993a: 200–208) in her study on communication in a Welsh geriatric hospital. She focused on the occurrence of greetings, inquiries about a patient's wellbeing, and other elements of 'phatic communion' (Malinowski 1923, Laver 1975, Coupland et al. 1992). She explores how these are used to prepare 'the commencement of the non-verbal routine' that is sure to follow. Grainger concludes that even though such instances of 'personal discourse' are a common component of opening phases, their ultimate goal is to get the care tasks on track.

Sachweh (2000: 262–263) in her study in a German eldercare facility took a more quantitative look at the opening phase. She analysed the occurrence of greeting sequences (both in openings and closings) in her data and found two regularities: First, the large majority of greeting exchanges were initiated by the care workers. In Sachweh's view, this is only partially explained by 'the general rule that the person who enters greets first'. An additional factor is that the care workers as 'agents of the institution' have a prerogative to the first turn. In part related to this, Sachweh's second finding is that more than half of the greeting sequences initiated by the care workers lacked a reply by the residents. This, according to Sachweh, shows that greeting in the context of eldercare is understood predominantly as a signal to frame the care process, rather than a phatic exchange.

Posenau's (2014: 77–88) findings largely confirm this. In his study, also in a German care context, he finds that the most common opening was a combined greeting + address turn by the care workers, used to wake up the residents and focus their attention on the upcoming activities. He also observes that a reply to this greeting was rather unusual, which he considers one reason why the care workers frequently repeated their greeting until they would be sure of a resident's interactional availability. After the greeting, some of the interactions move directly into the care routines; others do not contain a greeting at all. According to Posenau (2014: 83), this shows that the accomplishment of the care activities is given priority, to an extent that the care workers may even flout most basic social conventions. Posenau sees this as another indication of institutional asymmetries, allowing the care workers to shape an opening in any way they consider fit.

Before going into the analysis, a few specifics of the present data should be outlined. One is that we need to distinguish between those interactions that are initiated by a resident's nurse call and those that are not. The former constitute a minority of the cases, with only 12 openings that were clearly identifiable as following on a resident's call via the intercom. In various other cases, a preceding nurse call is recognisable on the recording and/or documented in the activity logs, but it remains ambiguous if the call was really made by the resident in question. As we will see, where a resident does open with a nurse call, this can have some crucial impact on the subsequent part of the interaction.

A second specific is that, unlike in other studies, the morning care activities in Edogawa Care are not necessarily the 'first contact' (see Weinhold 1997: 43) between a resident and a care worker on that day. As described in the methodology chapter (see section 3.1), the morning care is done by the night shift, which means that there may have been previous encounters between the participants during the night. This has likely implications for the design of an opening in that the participants, explicitly or not, may refer back to these earlier meetings when they 're-assemble' for the morning care activities. Also, as we have seen in the last example from the previous chapter (see excerpt 4.8), a care worker may have been in interaction with another resident in the same room and thus in physical proximity well in advance of the new exchange.

In order to get a closer idea of the structural properties of the opening phase, we start with one relatively prototypical example, presented in excerpt 5.1. It has been chosen because it contains all of the characteristic components that are commonly included in the openings of the sample. These are:

(1) a preparation phase, in advance of the verbal interaction (line 1),
(2) a summons (line 2),
(3) a greeting (line 3), and
(4) a clarification about the reasons for the encounter (starting in line 5).

Excerpt 5.1 (#14'1–8)

1	CW	((enters room, opens bed curtains))
2		LN-*sa:n*, LN-*san*
3		*ohayoo gozaimasu* Good morning.
4		(0.8)
5		*sorosoro okimasu ka:* Are you getting up?
6		(1.0)
7	Res	*soo desu ne:* Yes, you're right
8	CW	*un:* Uh-huh

Each of them will be discussed in turn, and further explored in comparison with other openings from the sample.

5.1.1 Preparations, summons, greeting

Like most of the interactions in the data, excerpt 5.1 starts with the care worker entering the room and making some minimal preparations prior to any verbal exchange. In the present case, she opens the resident's bed curtains, which is necessary, among other things, to establish visual contact between the two prospective interlocutors. In addition, the opening of the bed curtains serves to communicate to the resident that he (rather than the three other potential candidates in the room) is the next person to be attended to. Thus, a first important task that needs to be addressed at the very beginning of an opening is to determine and secure a partner for the upcoming exchange. While this holds true for most types of interactions, it seems particularly relevant in the present context, where there is usually more than one possible participant around.

The first one to speak in the excerpt is the care worker, in line 2. This is another common feature of the 107 interactions, no less than 102 of which have the care worker as first speaker. It suggests that there is some mutual understanding that the staff member should be the one to start the verbal exchange. This is largely in line with Sachweh's (2000) and Posenau's (2014) observations as discussed in this section's introduction, and seems to follow a more general principle of territoriality according to which the 'moving participant' first talks to the 'static participant' (Laver 1975: 226).

The care worker starts with calling the resident's name, which is the second common component of our openings. Apart from being an even more explicit specification of the resident to be attended to, this call with a vocative address term (see section 4.1) also works as a summons to ensure a resident's availability for the unfolding interaction. This resonates with Leech (1999: 108), who holds that two main functions of vocatives are addressee identification and summoning attention. The 'establishment of copresence' (Robinson 1998: 102) via an address term is particularly relevant in the present setting, given that many residents around this time of day/night are still asleep and thus not yet interactionally 'in play' (Schegloff 1968: 1086). In accord with Posenau's (2014) observations, the opening line thus frequently has a by-function as a wake-up call. An example is presented in excerpt 5.2.

In this exchange, the preparation phase consists of the care worker's entering the room and turning the resident's bed light on. Here, too, the verbal interaction starts with the care worker calling the resident's name, in line 2. Her lengthening of the honorific suffix *sa:n* plus the accompanying tapping at some of the resident's bed utensils underline the summons character of this (both verbal and

Excerpt 5.2 (#1'1–10)

1	CW	((enters room, light on))
2		FN-*sa:n* ((tapping [))
		FN-*san*
3	Res	[*aiai=*
4		=*ai*[*a*
5	CW	[FN-*san*
		FN-*san*
6		(0.6)
7	Res	(*a/ a:*)=
8	CW	=*ohayoo gozaima:su*
		Good morning
9	Res	*ohayo*
		Morning
10	CW	*un:*
		Uh-huh

non-verbal) call. The resident reacts with a few drowsy syllables (lines 3 and 4) that strongly suggest she has just been woken up. The pattern is repeated in lines 5 (care worker's call) and 7 (resident's semi-somnolent reaction).

After co-presence has been established in this way, the interactions in both excerpts proceed to the third component: the greeting phase. In both cases, the greeting is started by the care worker, which is another characteristic feature of the data. In total, 87 of the openings (81%) contain some sort of greeting activity, a mere three of which are initiated by the resident. In other words, the care worker is not only expected to initiate an interaction, as just described, but also to be the one who starts the greeting exchange. The former is a sequential consequence of the latter, as the verbal or non-verbal reaction of a resident to a care worker's summons transfers the responsibility for the relevant next action, the greeting, back to the care worker (see Schegloff 1968).

The most common greeting formula is *ohayoo gozaimasu* ('Good morning') and its informal variant *ohayo(o)* (see section 4.2.1), which occurs in 75 of the 107 interactions. Other greeting phrases that are sometimes used are *o-machidoo sama desu* and *o-matase shimashita* 'Sorry for making you wait' (see section 4.3.1), as well as the two apology expressions *gomen(nasai)* and *shitsurei shimasu*.

A noteworthy difference between the two excerpts is the resident's reaction to the care worker's greeting, which forms the first pair part (FPP) of an adjacency pair. Whereas in excerpt 5.2, the resident delivers the expected second pair part (SPP) *ohayo* in direct adjacency to the preceding FPP, in line 8, there is no such SPP in excerpt 5.1. Here, what follows the care worker's FPP is a pause of 0.8 seconds (line 4), after which the interaction moves on without a verbal reaction by the resident. This, too, is a common feature in the data: Of the 75 interactions with a care worker's *ohayo(o gozaimasu)* FPP, only 40 have

Excerpt 5.3 (#17'1–7)

1	CW	((enters room, opens bed curtains))
2		LN-*sa:n*
		LN-*san*
3		(1.3)
4		*ohayoo gozaimasu*
		Good morning
5		(1.8)
6		*ohayoo*
		Morning
7	Res	(°*ohayo*°)
		Morning

a clearly identifiable SPP by a resident. Again this concurs with Sachweh's (2000) and Posenau's (2014) findings, as described above.

As a result of the missing greeting SPP, the care workers frequently engage in some sort of prodding to elicit an appropriate response from a resident. One such example is presented in excerpt 5.3. Here, the care worker after entering the room and calling the resident's name starts a greeting sequence with *ohayoo gozaimasu* (line 4). When after a pause of 1.8 seconds there is still no reaction by the resident, the care worker expands the sequence by repeating her greeting (line 6). Note that she does so in a stylistically downgraded format, omitting the hyper-formal copula verb *gozaimasu*. Only after this second call does the resident deliver the requested SPP to complete the sequence. This way of eliciting a second pair part from a resident through repetition of the first pair part in a 'subsequent version' is a frequent feature throughout the data that will be discussed in more detail in chapter 7 (see section 7.3).

Another notable feature of greeting exchanges in the data is that they frequently end with what in conversation analysis is called a sequence closing third (SCT). This is an optional third turn delivered in response to a second pair part. In excerpt 5.2, for instance, the resident's greeting SPP in line 9 does not yet constitute the end of the sequence. Instead, it is followed by *un:* in line 10, a sequence closing third that functions as a sort of acknowledgment of receipt of the resident's reply. A closer analysis of this pattern, which is common also in various types of sequences outside the opening phase, will be provided in the next chapter (see section 6.1.2).

5.1.2 Reason for the encounter

The fourth key component of the openings is the reason for the encounter, corresponding to what in research on doctor–patient communication has been called 'reason for the visit' (ten Have 1991: 142) or 'accounting for the visit'

Excerpt 5.4 (#14'1–10)

1	CW	((enters room, opens bed curtains))
2		LN-*sa:n,* LN-*san*
3		*ohayoo gozaimasu* Good morning
4		(0.8)
5		*sorosoro okimasu ka:* Are you getting up?
6		(1.0)
7	Res	*soo desu ne:* Yes, you're right
8	CW	*un:* Uh-huh
9		(7.5, unlocks bedrails)
10		*hai, karada okoshite:* Okay, sit up

(Heritage and Robinson 2006). In excerpt 5.1, given here in slightly extended form as excerpt 5.4, this topic is brought up by the care worker in line 5 through asking the resident if she will be getting up. The care worker uses the term *sorosoro*, an adverb that expresses a speaker's assessment about the timeliness of something to happen. After a pause of one second, the resident in line 7 replies to the care worker's question in the affirmative, thus consenting to the suggested course of action. This is acknowledged by the care worker with a sequence closing third in line 8, which formally concludes the opening phase and moves the interaction on to the main stage. When the care worker speaks next in line 10, after a pause of 7.5 seconds used to make preparations for getting the resident out of bed, they are already 'at it'. The care activities have started.

As the data have been recorded during the morning care, the default reason for the encounter is getting a resident out of bed. Usually, it is the care worker who introduces this topic, varyingly as 'getting up' (*okiru*), 'getting dressed' (*kigaeru*), 'going to the toilet' (*toire iku*), or a combination of these. In excerpt 5.4, the issue is presented as a question that asks for the resident's consent with the suggested course of action (line 5). It is relatively quickly granted by the resident (line 7), though the preceding pause of one second suggests some hesitation. Such reluctance to agree with getting up can be even more pronounced, as is the case in excerpt 5.5.

This interaction, too, contains all the standard components of openings discussed so far: preparation (line 1), summons and greeting (lines 2 and 3), and the reason for the encounter, first put forward by the care worker in line 4.

Excerpt 5.5 (#3'1–20)

1	CW	((enters room))
2		FN-*san ohayoo gozaima*[*:su*
		FN-san good morning
3	Res	[*ohayo*
		Morning
4	CW	*okimasu yo*[*:*
		(We/you)'re getting up
5	Res	[*(nanji ima?)*
		What time now?
6	CW	*okiru jika:n*
		Time to get up.
7	Res	*nanji?*
		What time?
8		(0.3)
9	CW	°(*ro*)*kuji*°
		6 o'clock
10	Res	*un?*
		What?
11	CW	*rokuji:*
		6 o'clock
12	Res	*rokuji?*
		6 o'clock?
13	CW	*un*
		Uh-huh
14	Res	*un::,*
		Hmm::
15		(5.0, CW unlocks bedrails)
16		*rokuji ka=*
		6 o'clock you say
17	CW	=*un*
		Uh-huh
18		(0.4)
19		*hai, okimasu* [*yo*
		Okay, we're getting up
20	Res	[*hai*
		Okay

One difference to excerpt 5.4 is that in the present case, the care worker expresses the reason for her coming in a declarative rather than an interrogative format (also see section 6.1). In combination with the assertive discourse particle *yo*, this expresses her determination to see this matter through whether or not the resident will agree with it.

The resident reacts with a question about the time (line 5). She withholds her explicit consent at this point and instead brings up a new, though closely related, topic. Structurally speaking, she temporarily suspends the relevance of the care worker's FPP (line 4) by launching a new sequence with a new FPP. As first explored by Pomerantz (1984a), such 'requests for clarification' are a common way of framing so-called 'dispreferred' actions, such as, in the present case, the resident's reservations as to the care worker's statement to get her up.

The care worker's reply to the resident's new FPP deserves some special attention. Rather than giving her the factual time, the care worker tells the resident that it is *okiru jika:n*, 'time to get up' (line 6), thus reemphasising her determination to get the resident out of bed. Not satisfied with this sort of reply, obviously, the resident repeats her question in line 7. And this time, the care worker does provide the expected type of answer, though in a rather voiceless whisper that is difficult to understand (line 9). As a result, the resident in line 10 initiates what conversation analysts call a 'repair' sequence by indicating that she did not properly understand the care worker's previous utterance. The trouble persists even after the care worker's repetition of the time in line 11, which entails more repair work in lines 12 and 13.

Though at this point the time has been unambiguously clarified, the resident still seems unwilling to grant permission about getting up and address the pending FPP from line 4. Instead, she replies with a non-committal *un:* that expresses acknowledgment of the time as just reported by the care worker, but also shows her persisting reservations as to the suggested course of action.

In the meantime, the care worker is already making preparations for the upcoming care activities, as can be understood from the sound of the bedrails being unlocked (line 15). The resident once more repeats the time just told her (line 16), this time with the question particle *ka* attached, which frames her utterance as some sort of open soliloquy that expresses further hesitation. After confirming once more with a latched *un* in line 17, the care worker finally restates the reason for the encounter by proffering a new version of her previous FPP (line 19). It is preceded by *hai,* 'Okay', which signals the imminence of an upcoming task (see section 6.1.3). This time, the resident provides the requested SPP without any further delay, and even partially in overlap with the care worker's preceding turn. This officially concludes the opening phase by allowing the action to proceed to the tasks.

Excerpt 5.5 shows that a resident's consent in this 'negotiation process', as it has been called by Herzberger (1999: 38), is not always granted as easily as in the previous examples. In fact, the care worker's statement about getting up is followed by a longer insert of sequences about the time. These can be construed as an expression of disagreement, or at least hesitation, on the part of the resident. This entails some additional persuasion efforts by the care worker, as a result of which the opening phase draws longer than in the examples discussed so far. I have examined three similar excerpts from the data in more detail in an earlier article (Backhaus 2010). Important to note is that in all four cases, as in the majority of cases in general, the care workers eventually succeed in having things done their way.

One strategy to circumvent the risk of lengthy negotiations is to simply omit the reason for the encounter altogether and proceed right to the tasks. Such an example is presented in excerpt 5.6, the beginning of which has previously been given as excerpt 5.3. As described above, the interaction starts as usual, with the care worker entering the room and making preparations (line 1). Next, there is the care worker's summons (line 2) and greeting FPP (line 4), repeated in line 6 before the resident delivers the requested SPP in line 7. Rather than addressing the reason for the encounter now, however, the care worker moves straight on to the preparations of getting the resident out of bed (line 8, unlocking the bed rails). She does not make any direct mention of what is happening, let alone ask the resident if this is in line with what she would like to happen.

The resident's inquiry about the time and the ensuing repair sequence (lines 9–12) do not entail further talk about the reason for the care worker's coming either. Though the resident's main motivation for asking may be to elicit just such talk, the care worker's minimal response suggests that she is not willing

Excerpt 5.6 (#17'1–14)

1	CW	((enters room, opens bed curtains))
2		LN-*sa:n*
		LN-*san*
3		(1.3)
4		*ohayoo gozaimasu*
		Good morning
5		(1.8)
6		*ohayoo*
		Morning
7	Res	(°*ohayo*°)
		Morning
8		(10.0, CW unlocks bedrails)
9		(*nanji ima?*)
		What time now?
10	CW	*e?*
		What?
11	Res	*nan(###)*
		What
12	CW	*nanji? ima rokuji*
		What time? 6 o'clock
13		(9.0, preparations continue)
14		*hai,*
		Okay

to discuss the matter any further. Later, in line 14, when the care worker announces some imminent physical task with *hai*, 'Okay' (see section 6.1.3), it turns out that the opening phase has been concluded without any explicit reason for the encounter given. Facts have been established without words. Similar patterns of avoiding the business of compliance gaining have been described by Grainger (1993a: 203) and Posenau (2014: 85), suggesting that such strategies may be a common feature in care communication in general.

Sometimes, the reason for the encounter is brought up prior to the greeting. In excerpt 5.7, for instance, the issue is addressed directly after the summons (line 2), with the care worker asking 'Are you getting up?' in line 4. As the resident's attempt to reply is somewhat difficult to make out, the care worker repeats his question in line 6, partially still in overlap with the resident's previous turn. Most likely after some non-verbal indication by the resident in SPP position, the care worker reconfirms with *un* in line 8, directly after which he turns on the bed light.

The ensuing greeting sequence shows many of the common characteristics outlined so far: It is initiated by the care worker (line 10), replied to by the resident only after a subsequent version (lines 11–13), and completed by the care worker with a sequence closing third (line 14). What clearly differs from

Excerpt 5.7 (#52'1–14)

1	CW	((enters room))
2		LN-*sa:n*
		LN-*san*
3		(3.0)
4		*okiru?*
		Are you getting up?
5	Res	*effuheh*[*he*
		((groaning))
6	CW	[*okiru?*
		Are you getting up?
7		(0.5)
8		*un*
		Uh-huh
9		(1.2, light on)
10		*ohayoo*
		Morning
11		(1.7)
12		*ohayoo*
		Morning
13	Res	*nn ohayoo*
		m-morning
14	CW	*un*
		Uh-huh

the previous excerpts (and most other interactions of the sample) is that the greeting is delivered only after the subsequent course of action has been established. This reversed order of greeting and reason for the encounter shows the high importance of getting a resident's consent about proceeding with the morning care activities, and how this may suspend or at least postpone the more phatic activity of greeting.

5.1.3 Opening with nurse call

The openings discussed so far have been relatively similar in structure, starting with a care worker entering the room and making preparations for the subsequent interaction. Quantitatively speaking, this is by far the most common pattern, but it is not the only one. As previously mentioned, a smaller number of the cases are initiated by a resident's nurse call. As shown in excerpt 5.8, an opening may unfold in an entirely different way when this happens.

When the nurse call starts ringing in line 1, the care worker is still in the dayroom with another resident. Hearing the characteristic beep of the intercom, she quickly retrieves the room number of the calling resident from her mobile device and gets on her way. The first thing she does on entering the resident's room is turn the nurse call off. The verbal interaction starts with the care worker's (*o-*)*machidoo sama de:su* 'Sorry for making you wait' in line 3, which is both a greeting and a token of acknowledgment that the resident has been waiting. This second function makes it particularly feasible for nurse call openings, though it sometimes occurs in openings without a previous call, too.

The interaction continues with the resident asking the care worker to get him out of bed (line 4). The nurse replies in the affirmative (line 5) and after

Excerpt 5.8 (#83'1–9)

1	Res	((nurse call))
2	CW	((moves to resident's room, enters))
3		(*o-*)*machidoo sama de:su* Sorry for making you wait
4	Res	*suimasen okoshite itadakemasu ka=* Sorry, could you get me up?
5	CW	=*hai* Okay
6		(1.3)
7		*o-toire kimasu?* Are you going to the toilet?
8	Res	*hai* Yes
9	CW	*hai* Okay

a brief pause, asks the resident if he would like to go to the toilet (line 7). This is confirmed by the resident in line 8, and reconfirmed by the care worker with a sequence closing third in line 9, which marks the end of the opening phase.

The crucial difference to the excerpts discussed so far is that in the present case, the summons is not made by the care worker but by the resident. Despite being the first spoken line, the care worker's opening with (*o-*)*machidoo sama de:su* structurally is the second pair part (SPP) to an adjacency pair, the corresponding first pair part (FPP) of which is the resident's ringing of the nurse call. In this respect, this nurse call opening shows similarities with the summons–answer structure of openings in telephone calls as first observed in Schegloff's (1968) classic study. In both cases, the interactions are initiated by a non-verbal 'attention-getting device' in FPP position that comes from a machine but is triggered by a human.

The fact that it is the resident rather than the care worker who makes the summons and thus gains 'access to first position' (ten Have 1991: 146) has some non-trivial repercussions on the subsequent part of the opening. As the care worker's greeting in line 3 is in fact an SPP, the next one to speak is again the resident, and it is for him now to put forward the reason for the encounter: 'Sorry, could you get me up?' This is one of the few cases in the data where the resident rather than the care worker specifies what is to be done next.

The mechanism behind this can be explained in two ways. First, and obviously, the care worker cannot definitely know the reason for the encounter, as she has been called by the resident rather than come to him with some concern of her own. Second, as has just been shown, the fact that the summons comes from the resident effectively reverses the sequential roles of the participants at the beginning of the opening. As a result, when giving the reason for the encounter becomes a relevant next action, the resident qualifies as next speaker. This enables him to take the initiative in determining the subsequent flow of the actions, and thus assigns him a more proactive role than in most of the other openings.

In closing this section, let us take a brief quantitative look at the occurrence of the components described. Table 5.1 gives an overview of the 107 openings

Table 5.1 Occurrence of the four components in the opening phase

Components	Cases
Preparations, summons, greeting, reason	32 (30%)
Preparations, greeting, reason	30 (28%)
Preparations, greeting	18 (17%)
Preparations, reason	9 (8%)
Preparations, summons, greeting	9 (8%)
Preparations, summons, reason	7 (7%)
Preparations, summons	1 (1%)
Preparations, *hai*	1 (1%)
Total	107 (100%)

and the elements they contain (though not necessarily in that order). As can be seen, 30% of the openings have all four components, while another 28% do not have a summons. The third largest group is the 17% of interactions that lack a summons and a reason for the encounter. Three other sizeable groups are those that come without a greeting and a summons (8%), without a reason (8%), or without a greeting (7%).

The bird's eye view in Table 5.1 shows two things: First, the components that have been described as 'characteristic' at the beginning of the analysis indeed do feature in some way or other in most of the morning care openings. Yet, second, the great variety of combinations should clearly warn us against considering these components obligatory. In fact, the only component that is truly indispensable is the preparation phase, covering as it does the physical getting together of the participants that is essential for any kind of face-to-face interaction to occur. As to the four other components, we see that though there are some recognisable patterns, there is also much variation. In other words, the occurrence of these components is not prescribed by some unwritten rules, but determined by the participants on a case-by-case basis. The care workers do take the decisive role in this, but, as our final example has demonstrated, the residents have ways to influence the structure of an opening, too. The next section will show that this applies in a similar way to the organisation of the closings.

5.2 Closings

The interactional problem of closing a conversation was first discussed by Schegloff and Sacks in their seminal paper 'Opening up closings' (1973). Once the 'turn-taking machinery' is running, each delivered turn in an interaction by default generates the necessity for another turn to follow. If that next turn is not delivered as expected, this will not normally be heard as the end of the interaction, obviously, but as a silence within it, which needs to be accounted for some way or other. The main problem, according to Schegloff and Sacks (1973: 294–295), is 'how to organise the simultaneous arrival of the coconversationalists at a point where one speaker's completion will not occasion another speaker's talk', but at the same time 'will not be heard as some speaker's silence' either.

Schegloff and Sacks' analysis, again mainly based on telephone conversations, identifies a pre-closing phase that usually occurs at the end of 'topic talk' and provides an opportunity for the interlocutors to determine if all 'mentionables' have been addressed. This is most commonly done by items such as 'Okay' or 'Alright', delivered by one speaker in first pair part position and reciprocated by the other speaker with a similar item in second pair part position. Without either of them adding any new topic material, the 'pre-closing ceases to be "pre-"' (Schegloff and Sacks 1973: 309), and the exchange can proceed towards a quick termination.

An interaction ends with what the authors refer to as 'terminal exchanges'. These are good-byes or other farewell tokens, again occurring in adjacency pair format, which serve to remove the relevance of continued turn-taking. In other words, they put the turn-taking machinery to a halt, thus making possible the factual ending of an interaction through discontinuation of talk and physically disconnecting the participants. In the case of telephone conversations, this is achieved by hanging up. By contrast, when the participants are physically present, they will normally try to get out of reach of one another. An important feature of terminal exchanges is that they cannot be delivered just anywhere in the conversation, but only after the participants in the pre-closing have established the fact that there is no more topic talk to be done.

Schegloff and Sacks' framework was further developed by Button (1987), who focuses on one specific feature that frequently occurs towards the end of an interaction: moving out of closing. Working with a large sample of telephone conversations, he identifies various sequence types that are regularly used to suspend or cancel the trajectory of a running closing sequence. Button shows that moving out of closing may occur at different 'opportunity spaces' throughout the pre-closing and terminal exchange turns. In addition, he makes a basic distinction between minimal and drastic ways of moving out, depending on the relevance to move back into the closing in the turns that follow. If the closing can be re-initiated in the next turn, the move out is considered minimal. It is drastic if it cancels the immediate necessity to take up the suspended closing by introducing new topic material that is not relevant to the closing and will entail further topic talk.

Closing in medical settings has been examined by Heath (1986: 128–152) in his study of doctor–patient consultations in the UK. Unlike in telephone conversations, one main task the participants in such face-to-face encounters need to achieve is 'breaking each other's co-presence so that they are no longer interactionally or physically available' (Heath 1986: 129). In other words, they must find an appropriate way of getting out of eye and earshot. Using video data, Heath explores in great detail how the participants cooperate towards this goal through their verbal and non-verbal actions, particularly posture and gaze.

Weinhold (1997: 71–85) in her study on nurse–patient communication in a German hospital examined closings at the patients' rooms during morning and afternoon shifts. She found that closings in the former tended to be shorter and less complex, and frequently did not contain any terminal exchanges. She attributes this to the fact that patients and nurses know they will likely see each other again at least once during the next couple of hours. Given these circumstances, the lack of a terminal exchange can be seen as an indication of 'constant availability' (1997: 75) by the nurses, beyond the ending of the present encounter. By contrast, the last encounter of the afternoon shift will also be the participants' last encounter for the day. As Weinhold's data show, this requires a more explicit and sophisticated way of leave-taking, since the nurses will be no longer available for some time afterwards. This is also a relevant issue with respect to the closing phases of the present data, to which we will now turn.

5.2.1 Getting ready to leave

Unlike the openings as discussed in the previous section, all of which took place in the residents' rooms, the physical environment of the closings is more diverse. As described in chapter 3, there are various places where an interaction can come to an end. In total, we can distinguish four different locations. Most frequently, an interaction ends after a care worker has taken a resident to the toilet, has finished all necessary preparations there, and gets ready to leave. This type of closing occurs in over 60% of the cases. A second larger group of interactions end in a resident's room, either because the resident did not need to go to the toilet or does not need help with it, or because the participants have returned to the resident's room afterwards. Around 23% of the encounters end this way. Two less frequent types of closings occur in the hallway, when a resident is heading for the dayroom or the toilet (7.5%), and after arriving at the wash section at one end of the dayroom (6.5%). The figures are summarised in Table 5.2.

One general feature of the interactions is that there is a high likeliness of imminent follow-up encounters. In most cases, an interaction ends at a point where the morning care activities are not yet completed and will be resumed later on, either with the same care worker or with the second night shift staff. Rather than endings in a narrower sense, it may therefore be more appropriate to conceive of the closings as mere interruptions within a larger, yet unfinished course of activities that is going to be continued soon. As we will see in the analysis, this has some implications for the way the closings in the data are organised. This fact notwithstanding, all 107 cases qualify as closings in that the participants at least temporarily take leave of each other and thus 'break their co-presence' (Heath 1986).

The analysis starts with an example from the largest group of interactions: those ending at the toilet. It was chosen because it contains in a relatively straightforward way all of the basic complements of closings as they were first identified by Schegloff and Sacks (1973). In order to provide a broader view of the flow of events, excerpt 5.9 starts a few turns in advance of the beginning of the closing phase itself, when the participants have left the resident's room and are heading for the toilet.

Table 5.2 Places where closings occur

Place	Frequency
Toilet	67 (62.2%)
Room	25 (23.4%)
Hallway	8 (7.5%)
Dayroom	7 (6.5%)
Total	**107 (100%)**

Excerpt 5.9 (#83'87–99)

87	CW	*sotchi tomete morat°te ii desu ka°*
		Could you apply the brake on this side?
88		(10.0)
89	Res	*yoisho*
		((heave-ho))
90		(12.0)
91	CW	*ii desu ka?*
		Are you ready?
92		(0.7)
93		*daijoobu desu?=*
		Alright?
94	Res	*=ee, daijoobu desu=*
		Yes, alright
95	CW	*=hai, ja owatta[ra yonde kudasa:i*
		Okay, then please call when you have finished
96	Res	[*hai, arigatoo gozaimasu,*
		Yes, thank you
97		*suima[sen*
		and sorry
98	CW	[*ha:i*
		Okay
99		((leaves))

In line 87, the care worker asks the resident to apply the brake on one side of his wheelchair, most likely while she is doing the reverse side. This is followed by ten seconds of silence during which they make preparations to move the resident from his wheelchair to the toilet seat. The resident's next turn, in line 89, is a heave-ho token (see section 6.1.4), probably uttered at the moment he rises from the wheelchair. Another silence of 12 seconds follows, at the end of which it is safe to assume that the transfer from wheelchair to toilet has been completed.

The closing proper starts in line 91, with the care worker asking if everything is alright now. Getting no immediate reaction from the resident, she reformulates her question in a subsequent version in line 93. The resident confirms in line 94, thus acknowledging that in his view, all necessary preparations have been completed. The sequence from lines 91 to 94 thus has a pre-closing function in that it paves the way for the terminal exchange. However, in contrast to previous analyses of closings as discussed above, the pre-closing here is not designed to establish that all mentionables have been addressed; rather, it serves to confirm that all to-dos have been properly performed.

Noteworthy in this respect is the long silence that precedes the beginning of the pre-closing (line 90). Though due to the lack of video data we cannot know for sure what exactly is going on during these 12 seconds, it is obvious that the participants are working through some task here that neither affords nor entails any verbal exchange. It is only after this task has been completed that the talk is resumed. This means that the participants in the pre-closing do not primarily work towards stopping the 'turn-taking machinery' by passing up opportunities for new topic talk, as has been shown by Schegloff and Sacks (1973), and others. Contrarily, the machinery is on hold anyway, and the participants re-launch it only to close the interaction in an orderly fashion. In order to do so, they need to make sure that all things that need to be done have been adequately dealt with at this point, and that is where language comes back in. In other words, in the present setting, it is primarily the contents of the tasks – not the contents of the talk – that determine the course of the interaction and when it is due to be closed.

The final component in excerpt 5.9 is the terminal exchange, which starts in line 95. The care worker briefly acknowledges the resident's confirmation and then goes on to announce her imminent leave by reminding him to push the nurse call button when finished (line 95). This is confirmed by the resident in lines 96 and 97 with a token of gratitude and an apology. The care worker acknowledges on her part, and leaves directly afterwards.

In contrast to terminal exchanges in most previous studies, there is no identifiable farewell token. Instead, the beginning of the sequence is designed as a request by the care worker in first pair part position, and its acceptance by the resident as a second pair part. In the data, this is in fact the standard pattern for terminal exchanges at the toilet. As can be seen, it is effective in cancelling the relevance of more turn-taking and bringing the interaction to a close, with a ratified departure by the care worker that will quickly break off the communication channel.

72 interactions, or about two thirds of all cases, contain an identifiable terminal exchange FPP. Except for one case, to which we will turn later, all terminal exchanges are initiated by the care workers. The great majority are designed as a request – most frequently a reminder to a resident to push the nurse call button when finished. In interactions that end at a resident's room or in the hallway, care workers occasionally make other requests, for example asking a resident to briefly wait in front of an occupied toilet or wheel themselves to the washing section to put in their dentals. These are relatively rare cases though, which make up only 13 of the 64 requests.

Only three interactions include terminal exchanges with standard farewell tokens: *o-yasumi*, an abbreviated version of *o-yasumi nasai* 'Good night', used in one of the rather exceptional cases where a care worker has put a resident back to bed after returning from the toilet (#47); *itte kuru* 'Bye' or, literally, 'I'll be right back', which a care worker says to a resident on leaving for an incoming nurse call (#57); and *dewa dewa* 'So long', which is how a care worker takes leave of a relatively independent resident after getting her dressed and suggesting that she should now relocate to the toilet (#66).

In addition, there are three cases in which completion assessments such as *ato daijoobu ne* 'Everything else okay then?' (#46) initiate a terminal exchange. Finally, two terminal exchange FPPs are designed as arrangements that explicitly refer to a subsequent encounter of the two participants during the same shift: *roku ji kuru wa* 'I'll be back at 6 o'clock' (#34) and *ja ato de iku kara* 'So I'll come later then' (#99). In both cases, the care worker parts from the residents at their room. The data are summarised in Table 5.3.

Of the 72 terminal exchange FPPs, 48 continue with a corresponding SPP. In the overall majority of cases, this is a token of acknowledgment such as *hai*, *un*, or sometimes *e:* (#49) or *a:* (#48). These are occasionally followed by a token of gratitude (#83, see excerpt 5.9) or an apology (#10). A somewhat exceptional SPP is *itterasshai*, produced in reply to the previously mentioned *itte kuru* FPP (#57). This is the only instance in the data where a genuine *goodbye* token occurs in SPP position. Finally, there is one case where a care worker's terminal exchange FPP is openly rejected by a resident, which leads into a moving out of closing. We will get back to this example at the end of the section (see excerpt 5.15).

As previously mentioned, a terminal exchange is normally initiated by the care worker. The only exception in the data is presented in excerpt 5.10 – another ending that occurs at the toilet. It starts with the last task before the

Table 5.3 Occurrence and types of terminal exchange FPPs

Type or terminal exchange	Frequency
- Requests	64 (59.8%)
- Standard farewell tokens	3 (2.8%)
- Completion assessments	3 (2.8%)
- Arrangements	2 (1.9%)
No terminal exchange	35 (32.7%)
Total	**107 (100%)**

Excerpt 5.10 (#98'225–234)

225	CW	*hai FN-san suwarinaoshima*[*:su*
		Okay, FN-san, I'll sit you down again
226	Res	[*hai*
		Okay
227		(3.0)
228		*zettai kite ne:*
		Do come back, will you?
229	CW	*haiiyo:*
		Yeah
230		(1.0)
231		*kimasu yo*
		I will
232		(0.4)
233	Res	*hai*
		Okay
234		((leaves))

closing – making the resident sit down on the toilet seat. The action is announced by the care worker in line 225, confirmed by the resident in line 226, and performed during the three seconds that follow. Line 228 is the FPP of the terminal exchange and, as in the majority of cases, it is designed as a request. One substantial difference to all other terminal exchange FPPs is that this is a request made by the resident, not by the care worker. The care worker on her part provides the corresponding SPP, an acknowledgment of the request in line 229.

The temporary reversal of the turn structure here achieves two things. First, it designates the resident as the one to assess that all to-dos have been done, which, second, enables her to make a request herself rather than merely react to one made by the caregiver. The resident's deviation from the common, more passive pattern may arise from the fact that, as she complains at the beginning of the exchange, she had already been waiting for a rather long time when calling for the morning care to start. Her explicit request for the care worker's quick return can be understood as an attempt to avoid such trouble when she calls next. In a way similar to the nurse call opening discussed at the end of the previous section (see excerpt 5.8), the reversed turn structure allows the resident to more substantially influence the course and timing of the actions. And, coincidence or not, the activity log of that day shows that the care worker does come back directly after the resident's next nurse call.

5.2.2 Leave without verbal acknowledgment

So far, we have seen that the terminal exchange plays an important role in the closing of the morning care interactions. However, it must not be forgotten that there is a substantial number of cases that end without any recognisable terminal exchange at all. As could be seen in Table 5.3, this applies to almost one third of the interactions in the sample. We will now take a closer look at how the closing is organised in such cases.

One pattern that is frequently observable for interactions without a terminal exchange is an ending on *hai*, 'Okay' (see section 6.1.3) or a similar token of acknowledgement at the end of the last task. An example is presented in excerpt 5.11, in which we join the resident and the care worker on their way

Excerpt 5.11 (#44'26–33)

26		(17.0, to toilet)
27	CW	°*yoisho*° (1.5)
		((heave-ho))
28		*hai,*
		Okay
29		(16.0)
30		*hai oroshima:su*
		Okay, I let you down
31		(2.5)
32		*hai,*
		Okay
33		((leaves))

to the toilet. Arrival there coincides with a whispered heave-ho token by the care worker in line 27, followed by *hai,* in line 28, which can be taken as an announcement of the beginning of the next task, most likely the resident's move from wheelchair to toilet. The largest part of this task is performed during the 16 seconds of silence that follow. After everything has been prepared, the care worker in line 30 announces that she will now sit the resident down on the toilet. Completion of this task is acknowledged with another *hai,* which marks the end of the verbal interaction. The care worker leaves directly afterwards.

The closing in this interaction works entirely without terminal exchange tokens. Instead, it ends with a simple completion marker of the task that just happens to be the last task. This suggests some mutual understanding between the participants that once this 'last task' has been performed, an interaction may in principle be terminated any time without further verbal ado. Again we see the predominance of the tasks and how they control the talk to be done, or left undone.

An additional factor that may contribute towards a 'wordless' departure by the care worker is the very intimate toilet situation that is just about to start here and that calls for utmost privacy, including a maximally quick and non-intrusive retreat by the care worker. In addition, we should not forget that there will most likely be a follow-up encounter directly after the resident has finished her toilet use. This may be another reason why the participants consider a terminal exchange unnecessary, or inappropriate even.

In some cases, the line between termination and temporary suspension is even more difficult to draw. An example is presented in excerpt 5.12, which is from an

Excerpt 5.12 (#25'43–52)

43		(11.0, out of toilet, to wash section in dayroom)
44	CW	LN-*san kao aratte* LN-san, wash your face
45	Res	*hai* Okay
46	CW	*hai* Okay
47		(8.0)
48		*ha,* (0.5) *ireru?* Dentals, put them in?
49		(1.5)
50		*ne:,* Right?
51		(4.5)
52		((leaves))

exchange that ends in the dayroom. The care worker has just wheeled the resident back from the toilet, and the two are now heading for the dayroom. When they arrive at the wash section, the care worker instructs the resident to wash her face (line 44) and asks if she would like to insert her dentals (line 48). She self-replies to this question in line 50, probably after some non-audible reaction by the resident. After staying nearby for another 4.5 seconds (no audible movement of feet or change of background noise), she leaves, moves through the hall, and then goes briefly back to the toilet before returning to the dayroom.

The most likely reason why the closing in this excerpt occurs without a terminal exchange is that the care worker knows she will get back to the resident very soon. And indeed, the activity log shows that she returns to the wash section after less than a minute, handing the resident her toothpaste. This illustrates that the methodological decision to consider the interaction closed at this point is somewhat arbitrary, and not necessarily in line with the participants' understanding of the situation. Assuming that the care worker knew she would be leaving only temporarily and thus did not regard the interaction as closed in the first place, delivery of a terminal exchange token at this point would appear much more unnatural than its absence.

5.2.3   *Moving out*

A final characteristic to be discussed here is the temporary suspension of a running closing sequence, commonly known as moving out of closing (Button 1987). There are 13 interactions in the data whose closing sequence shows this phenomenon. In the majority of them, ten in total, it is the care worker who initiates the moving out. Here, too, we can recognise the predominance by the representatives of the institution to determine the course of action. In order to get a better understanding of the moving out mechanisms, we will look at three examples in more detail.

Excerpt 5.13 is a sequence where the moving out of closing occurs after the first pair part of the terminal exchange (line 20). It is another ending at the toilet. The excerpt starts with the care worker's completion marker of the final task in line 18, followed by the standard 'when finished push button' request that constitutes the first pair part of the terminal exchange. However, instead of waiting for an acknowledgement by the resident – or calling for one, or just leaving without – the care worker attaches a reminder to the resident. She tells her that she might have to wait for some time after calling, as many other residents are getting up now, too (lines 22 and 25). The resident reacts with an apology (line 27), acknowledged by the care worker with a sequence closing third in line 28.

The care worker's reminder most likely refers back to past incidents regarding the resident's dissatisfaction with waiting times after a nurse call, some of which are documented in the recordings of the previous days. Incidentally, it is the same resident who in excerpt 5.10 reminded a (different) care worker to come back quickly when called for. The resident's reputation of being unwilling to

Excerpt 5.13 (#30'18–28)

18	CW	°*hai*°
		Okay
19		(2.3)
20		*owattara oshite ne:*
		Push when you've finished
21		(1.3)
22		*FN-san de mina* [*ima junban ni okiteru kara:,*
		FN-*san*, and everyone is getting up now in turn,
23	Res	[(*a*)
		Uh
24		(0.6)
25	CW	*narashite mo sugu korenai kara ne:*
		so even if you call we cannot come directly
26		(2.3)
27	Res	(*suima*)*sen*
		Sorry
28	CW	*u:n* ((leaving))
		Uh-huh

wait may be the main reason why the care worker finds it necessary to deviate from the ordinary closing structure and insert a preventive 'call not to call' at this stage. A direct comparison of excerpts 5.10 and 5.13 thus brings home the strategic importance of closings in shaping the post-closing developments.

A closer look at excerpt 5.13 also shows that the care worker's moving out of closing in line 20 substantially changes the trajectory of the sequence. Instead of a quick completion of the terminal exchange, the turn-taking machinery is reinitiated. This can be understood from the resident's backchannelling in line 23, as well as from the rather long pause of 2.3 seconds in line 26, which opens up after the care worker has finished her reminder, in expectation of a reaction by the resident. It is only after this reaction has been delivered, in line 27, that the interaction is brought to a close, incidentally without any new or recycled terminal exchange material. As can be understood from the background noise, the care worker at this point is already on her way out of the toilet room.

In the next example, moving out of closing occurs after the second pair part of the terminal exchange. Excerpt 5.14 is from an interaction that ends at the resident's room. The structure at the beginning of the excerpt can be sketched as follows: care worker's announcement of the end of the final task (line 143), resident's confirmation and expression of gratitude (line 144), care worker's completion assessment (see Table 5.3) as first pair part of the terminal exchange (lines 145–146), and resident's acknowledgment in second pair part position (line 147). This formally completes the closing sequence and should provide for a direct departure by the care worker.

Excerpt 5.14 (#10'143–154)

143	CW	*hai:=* Okay
144	Res	*=hai, arigatoo* [*gozaimasu* Okay, thank you
145	CW	[*hai, ja, ato=* Okay, then please
146		*=onegai shi*[*ma:su* do the rest by yourself
147	Res	[*hai, suimasen* Yes, thank you
148		(1.6)
149		*denki* The light
150		(0.5)
151	CW	*a, ja: keshitokima*[*ssu* Oh, I'll turn it off then
152	Res	[*hai, suima*[*sen* Yes, thank you
153	CW	[*hai* Okay
154		((arranges things in the room, leaves))

However, the interaction is reopened with a moving out of closing by the resident, who after a brief intermission reminds the care worker that she still needs to turn off the light (line 149). As can be understood from the audio data, the care worker at this point has already turned away from the resident. The resident's call thus literally catches her 'on the way out'. This unexpected turn of events is reflected in the care worker's reply in line 151, which starts with a 'change-of-state token' (Heritage 1984b, Sudo 2005) that shows her surprise. She assures the resident that she will take care of the light as requested, which is acknowledged by the resident in line 152, and reconfirmed by the care worker in line 153. These three final turns form a new terminal exchange – which has become necessary after the resident's moving out of closing has cancelled the validity of the previous one. Noteworthy here again is the dominance of the tasks: If some of the to-dos remain to be done, this warrants a reopening of an interaction even after it has already been formally closed.

The two examples discussed so far qualify for what Button (1987) has characterised as minimal moving out of closing. We will conclude this section with an example of a more drastic suspension of a closing sequence. Excerpt 5.15 is another ending at the toilet, which starts while the resident and the care worker are still engaged in topic talk about the appropriate use and misuse of

Excerpt 5.15 (#97'110–122)

110	Res	*tsukawanakya* [*son datte*
		As though you'd lose money if you didn't use it
111	CW	[*u::*[*n*
		Uh-huh
112	Res	[*omotte hito iru yo*
		That's what some people think
113		*chotto matte ne kore kara hajimaru*
		Hold on, it's about to start
114	CW	*un, yonde kudasa*[*i*
		Yeah, please call
115	Res	[*ii, datte, warui wa=*
		Oh no that's no good
116		*=sekkaku matte*[*te mora* (##)
		you (could be) waiting
117	CW	[*un, daijoobu yo* ((opening door))
		Yeah, no problem
118	Res	*kyuukei ni naru no mo, anata* [*ga*
		and it's going to be a break, for you
119	CW	[*ndaijoobu daijoobu*
		No problem no problem
120	Res	*soo?*
		Really
121	CW	*un*
		Yeah
122	Res	*suimasen, onegai shimasu* ((while CW is leaving))
		Sorry ((in-advance gratitude formula))

toilet paper. All necessary preparations are completed at this point, and the closing seems close ahead. It is just then that the resident asks the care worker to stay during her toilet use, which, as she announces, is just about to start (line 113).

The care worker kindly declines this offer (line 114). She does so by proffering *un* as a token of 'weak agreement' (Pomerantz 1984a) before annulling the resident's suggestion with the standard reminder to call when finished. While this could make for a potential pre-closing or terminal exchange, the resident reacts with another attempt to encourage the care worker to stay (lines 115–116). She does so partially in overlap with the care worker's previous turn, in an attempt to avert the imminent closing before it can materialise. As she now tries to explain, additional time spent waiting at the toilet without any immediate task to do may be a welcome opportunity for the care worker to take a break (line 118).

The care worker, however, obviously not willing to stay any longer than necessary with the resident in this situation, keeps declining the offer (lines 117 and 119). Here, too, she uses tokens of acknowledgment like *un* to soften her rejection, while insisting that it is *daijoobu* 'no problem' for her to go without the break. While saying this, she is already physically preparing to leave, as can be understood from her opening the toilet door in line 117. When she declines a fourth time, after a final call for confirmation by the resident (lines 120 and 121), she is already moving along outside the toilet room, as can be understood from the changed background noise. The 'deserted' resident finally concedes and closes the interaction with a token of apology, combined with a request to the care worker to come back later. At this point, her voice already sounds considerably far off.

Interesting about this excerpt is that the physical closing seems to proceed at a faster pace than the verbal closing. While the resident's moving out of closing is an attempt to postpone the end of the interaction, the care worker is eager to finish things up as soon as possible. The suggested 'break' with the toileting resident obviously does not seem as appealing to her as it does to the resident. That is why she tries to accelerate the held-up closing by starting to break the co-presence even before this has been ratified through the talk. In other words, two things that usually happen in succession – first, finish the talk, then break the communication channel – here happen at the same time. This also adds a certain hurriedness to the situation, to which we will return in chapter 7.

5.3 Discussion

This chapter has approached the interactions of the sample from their two endpoints: the openings, through which the participants get the morning care activities on track, and the closings, which bring the interactions to a coordinated and mutually ratified ending. With respect to the former, we have seen that there are some clearly identifiable components that the participants work through in advance of the main morning care activities. These include a preparation phase, a summons and a greeting, and a clarification of the reason for the encounter. Even though not all of these ingredients necessarily occur in each interaction, the analysis has shown that they demarcate a main path that largely shapes the trajectory of the openings.

Most essential, and in fact indispensable, is the preparation phase, in which the care worker enters a resident's room and moves 'within reach'. Given that most of the residents' rooms are four-bed rooms, a care worker in this phase must communicate to a resident that it is her or him rather than one of the three roommates who will be attended to. A crucial step in this identification process is the care worker's physical act of opening that resident's bed curtains, which, in a way, also officially opens up the interactional curtain.

The identification is verbally complemented by a care worker's summons and greeting. These two components frequently occur in direct succession, and in some cases fulfil the by-function of a wake-up call. The summoning is commonly done using a resident's first or last name, sometimes in repetition, and often with a lengthening of the person honorific *san* into *sa:n* . With respect to the findings from chapter 4, the frequent calling of a resident at this stage of the interaction may be an additional factor for the high frequency of vocative terms of address in the speech of the care workers (see section 4.1).

The most common greeting is *ohayoo gozaimasu* or just *ohayoo* '(Good) morning'. In the majority of cases, the greeting exchange is initiated by the care workers, and not necessarily reciprocated by the residents. This may entail some sort of prodding through subsequent versions of the greeting, which has been exemplified in excerpt 5.3. An interaction may also proceed without a greeting, particularly if there has been a previous encounter between the participants. This point was confirmed in one of the study sessions, where the care workers agreed that they considered a greeting unnecessary if they had met a resident 'only ten minutes before'.

The main reason for a care worker's coming is to get the resident out of bed. As the residents are not always willing to grant their consent with this, negotiations may be necessary before the interaction can move on to the main part. The line here between convincing and coercing (Candlin and Roger 2013: 76) is often difficult to draw. Sometimes, the care workers choose to take a 'shortcut' by omitting the reason for the encounter, and after the greeting proceed directly to the tasks. Asked about this point, the care workers said they would normally try to get consent from all 'alert persons' (*shikkari sareteru kata*), and would decide so on a case-by-case basis. Where compliance is asked for, the care workers eventually succeed in getting things done as requested. This is very much in line with Herzberger's (1999: 38) observations from an Austrian care institution.

The analysis of the closings has shown that there are both differences and similarities with previous research. Perhaps the greatest difference in comparison with the data analysed by Schegloff and Sacks (1973) arises from the fact that long silences during the morning care activities are normal, and do not seem to be considered an accountable interactional problem by the participants. Unlike Schegloff and Sacks' telephone conversations, we are not dealing with 'the problem of closing a conversation that ends a state of talk'. Rather, resident and care worker find themselves in what Schegloff and Sacks (1973: 325) characterise as 'a continuing state of incipient talk', in a similar way to 'members of a household in their living room, employees who share an office, passengers together in an automobile, etc.'. This has some crucial implications for the design of the closings in the present data. As the analysis of excerpt 5.9 has exemplified, the turn-taking machinery is frequently on hold during the morning care activities. It does not have to be stopped but needs to be re-started for the sole purpose of bringing it to an end. We could compare this to a computer in sleep mode, which cannot be shut down unless it is 'woken up' once more.

The main issue to be addressed in a closing is to determine whether all tasks have been completed at this stage. This means that the appropriate end of an interaction is mainly determined by and coincident with the end of the task work. Rather than agreeing that all 'mentionables' have been mentioned, the participants need to establish that all 'to-dos' have been done. This indicates the high relevance of the tasks during the morning care interactions, to which we will come back on various occasions throughout the following chapters.

The quantitative analysis has shown that two thirds of the interactions end with an identifiable terminal exchange FPP. Except for one case, it is always delivered by the care worker, and not necessarily reciprocated by the resident. The most common type of terminal exchange FPP is a request to call via intercom when finished, while more prototypical farewell tokens are extremely rare. This, too, testifies to the task-oriented nature of the encounter, but, as I learned during one of the study sessions, it also relates to a security issue. The care workers said that the 'when finished push button' phrase to them was important to make sure that the residents would not try to stand up from the toilet by themselves, as this could easily result in falls.

While it may at first seem strange that there are a sizeable number of interactions that come to an end without any terminal exchange, we must keep in mind that the participants know they are likely to see each other again fairly soon. In some cases, as shown in excerpt 5.12, it is only a matter of seconds until they cross paths next. In this respect, it may be more in line with the participants' understanding to regard their encounters as interrupted rather than closed. Asked about this point, the care workers showed a high awareness of the problem of such multi-encounters, explaining that they would often go for an extra farewell round at the very end of their shift to explicitly say good-bye to the residents one last time.

As the last part of the analysis has shown, the sample also includes a number of cases where the participants move out of a running closing sequence. This, too, is more frequently initiated by the care workers, though the residents occasionally 'move out' as well. The three examples we have explored demonstrate the interactional difficulties of coordinating the physical with the verbal leave-taking. This echoes Robinson (2001: note 4), who in a study on doctor–patient interactions observed that closing includes not only 'the termination of talk', but also 'termination of copresence'. This latter 'cannot be accomplished instantaneously (compared to, for example, hanging up a phone)', which substantially 'complicates the activity of closing because as long as people are copresent they are available to each other for further interaction'.

There is some possibility that this lingering co-presence of the participants after the terminal exchange, as for example in excerpt 5.14, will make it easier in such settings to move out of closing even after the would-be 'last word' has been said. As the final excerpt has shown, the participants may address this problem by starting to break off their co-presence while the verbal exchange is still under way.

The analysis of both the openings and closings demonstrates that it is largely the care workers who determine the interactional flow. They are the ones who 'pick' their partner, open the verbal interaction, launch a greeting, and call for a reply to it. They also initiate the terminal exchange, and expand or accelerate a running closing sequence. Similar observations have been made by Staples (2015) in a recent study on nurse–patient interactions in a US hospital.

However, we have also seen that there are cases where the residents manage to get a stronger grip on the unfolding of an exchange. Of note in this respect are the examples presented in excerpts 5.8 and 5.10, where a simple reversal of the turn structure provides for a much higher agency by the residents in determining how the action is to progress. A similar though less 'successful' case is described in Engbersen's (2013: 30–35) study of Dutch elderly care services. Exceptional as they may be, these examples illustrate that resident–staff interactions in Edogawa Care are not entirely pre-determined by the power asymmetries between the two groups, but that these asymmetries are subject to negotiation in the interactional give and take.

6 Talk at work

Having examined the beginnings and endings of morning care encounters, this chapter deals with the middle and main part, during which the physical tasks of the 'bed and body work' (Gubrium 1975: 125) are performed. This phase makes up the longest portion of an interaction by far and provides the participants with ample opportunities to talk – or remain silent – as they work through the tasks. But what exactly happens during this phase and how?

As described in section 2.2, one characteristic of care communication is that it is highly task-oriented while at the same time frequently interspersed with stretches of apparently unrelated 'homileic discourse' (Ehlich and Rehbein 1980: 343). The present data add to the evidence that resident–staff communication in eldercare, as in many other institutional settings, is both task work and talk work. The analysis presented in this chapter explores how each of the two elements needs to be properly addressed by the participants if they are to accomplish what they came for.

Previous researchers of communication in institutional settings have made a basic distinction between two types of talk, most commonly referred to as 'transactional talk' and 'relational talk'. Transactional talk is talk predominantly concerned with the institutional tasks, whereas relational talk is not directly related to the business at hand and includes what is more popularly known as 'small talk' (Coupland 2000). The two types of talk have been studied in various institutional environments, most commonly service encounters (Coupland and Ylänne-McEwen 2000, Kuiper and Flindall 2000, McCarthy 2000, Placencia 2004, Ylänne-McEwen 2004, Toerien and Kitzinger 2007, Félix-Brasdefer 2015, Taylor 2016), but also workplace interactions (Holmes 2000, Koester 2004) and healthcare settings (Beck and Ragan 1995, Ragan 2000, Major and Holmes 2008: 76, Menz and Plansky 2014).

In the context of institutional eldercare, a distinction has been made between those elements of speech that directly relate to a running care task and those that are not primarily motivated by the concurrent action line. For instance, Wagnild and Manning (1985) in their study of geriatric long-term care facilities in the US distinguish between 'procedural' and 'non-procedural' conversation. In a more recent study, Carpiac-Claver and Levy-Storms (2007) code staff–resident mealtime interactions into 'instrumental communication' and 'affective communication'. Ward et al. (2008) in their research in British dementia care classify their data into 'task-based' and 'social or relationship oriented' interactions. With respect to topic choice, Onoda (2014, 2016c) in his study of Japanese home help communication makes a basic distinction between task-related and non-task related topics (plus an intermediate category, which shows that this difference is not necessarily a clear-cut one), while Posenau (2014) in his research on German dementia care explores what he calls 'care-remote' topics and how they concur with the care activities. In a similar way, Engbersen (2013) in her Dutch data distinguishes between 'bound' and 'unbound' topics.

While most previous studies agree that relational talk is a non-obligatory component of institutional encounters, they also emphasise its favourable effects in smoothing the overall 'flow of discourse' (Félix-Brasdefer 2015: 184), which may temporarily even out the institutional asymmetries. For instance, in the context of gynaecological exams, Ragan (1990, 2000) has shown how elements of verbal play and extra-medical self-disclosure can contribute to a more equal relationship between doctor and patient, with potentially positive medical outcomes, too. This being the case, Ragan (2000: 270) contends that small talk is certainly 'not smaller' than any other type of talk. In a similar vein, Coupland (2000: 22) holds that in the context of communication with older people, small talk can be 'an important human and even medical resource', which clearly challenges 'the presumed "smallness" of small talk'.

One problem that has increasingly been explored in previous research is the sequential coordination of the transactional and relational elements of talk. In a study of workplace interactions, Koester (2004: 1415) explores how and at what points relational talk gets 'fitted in-between the transactional phases' of an interaction. Félix-Brasdefer (2015: 191) in his research in a supermarket deli demonstrates that shifts between the two modes of talk do not occur randomly, but are 'systematically synchronised according to the demands of the interaction, changing from transactional to relational talk to balance both the institutional orientation and the interpersonal demands for future transactions'. Toerien and Kitzinger's (2007) micro-analysis of an exchange in a beauty salon brings home the organisational problems of such shifts, particularly when they are to be performed in a maximally non-interruptive way. We will come back to this point in the course of the discussion.

Informed by previous approaches, this chapter makes a basic distinction between task talk and non-task talk. Task talk is defined here as all parts of the verbal exchange directly relating to some task that has just been, is being, or is about to be performed. Non-task talk, on the other hand, includes all those bits of talk that are not immediately related to the care tasks. Functionally speaking, task talk is essentially talk *for* getting things done, while non-task talk is talk *while* getting things done.

The analysis starts with a closer look at task talk, the basic components it consists of, and how they 'work' in interaction. The second part of the chapter examines non-task talk. A quantitative analysis identifies the most frequent topics residents and staff talk about and identifies differences in the topic preferences of the two groups. The third part focuses on shifts between task and non-task talk and the interactional difficulties such shifts entail.

6.1 Task talk

This section provides a basic overview of the various types of task talk that come with, and are in fact closely linked to, the care tasks. To be discussed are different forms of control acts (section 6.1.1), the structure of inquiry sequences (section 6.1.2), the functioning of the task transition marker *hai*, (section 6.1.3), and the use of heave-hoes and how they verbalise and coordinate physical activities (section 6.1.4). In addition, we will see that it is quite common for long stretches of silence to open up between these task-related elements of speech (section 6.1.5).

6.1.1 Control acts

One frequent component of task talk, and arguably the 'most central communicative action' (Posenau 2013: 77) during the morning care activities overall, is making directives, requests, and suggestions about what needs to be done next. Following Ervin-Tripp et al. (1990), I will use the summarising term 'control acts' to refer to this type of task talk. The term is understood here in a relatively straightforward way as referring to all types of speech acts that 'attempt to get someone to do something' (Vine 2004: 27).

Control acts have been extensively studied in interaction with and among children (Garvey 1975, Goodwin 1980, 1988, Wood and Gardner 1980, Wootton 1981, Ervin-Tripp et al. 1990, Sealey 1999, Kobayashi 2001, Craven and Potter 2010, Aronsson and Cekaite 2011, Goodwin and Cekaite 2013, Takada and Endo 2015, Nguyen and Nguyen 2016). As for institutional settings, researchers have examined control acts at the workplace (Weigel and Weigel 1985, Pufahl Bax 1986, J.S. Smith 1992, Vine 2004, Saito 2011, Mondada 2014), in service encounters (Aoyama 2002, Vinkhuyzen and Szymanski 2005, Kuroshima 2010, Sorjonen and Raevaara 2014, Bataller 2015, Li and Ma 2016), in the classroom (Wilkinson and Calculator 1982, Holmes 1983, Ellis 1992, Dalton-Puffer 2005, Riesco Bernier 2008), in doctor–patient interaction (Aronsson and Rundström 1989, West 1990, Harris 2003, Curl and Drew 2008), and in care for intellectually disabled persons (Finlay et al. 2008, Antaki and Kent 2012, Antaki and Crompton 2015). In addition, a handful of studies are now available that look at control acts in eldercare settings (Herzberger 1999, Lindström 2005, Heinemann 2006, Yamazaki et al. 2007, Marsden and Holmes 2014, Tachikawa 2015, Jansson 2016).

Starting with a seminal paper by Ervin-Tripp (1976), many earlier studies have sought to identify the formal and functional characteristics of control acts and how they come to be understood the way they are. Related to this, it has been examined how control acts can be mitigated or aggravated through various morphosyntactic and pragmatic devices (e.g., Linde 1988, Jones 1992) and how this may cross-culturally differ (e.g., Blum-Kulka et al. 1989, Fukushima 2003, Flöck 2016). Many previous studies have done so with reference to Brown and Levinson's (1987) politeness framework, according to which control acts harbour intrinsic threats to a hearer's face.

In research within the conversation analytical paradigm, a parallel interest developed in examining control acts as dispreferred actions (Pomerantz 1984a, Schegloff 2007: 81–96). Apart from studying how different syntactic formats can express different degrees of 'entitlement' to make a request (Lindström 2005, Heinemann 2006, Curl and Drew 2008, Craven and Potter 2010, Antaki and Kent 2012), there has been growing awareness of the 'sequential context' (Taleghani-Nikazm 2006) of control acts, including how they are prepared (e.g., Pufahl Bax 1986), received (e.g., Harris 2003), and accompanied by non-verbal actions (e.g., Rauniomaa and Keisanen 2012).

Likely the most common way to verbally communicate a control act in Japanese – and, in any case, the most frequent way appearing in my data – is through constructions with a verb in the *-te* form, a non-finite continuous verb form that is commonly combined with *kudasai* 'please' to formulate a request. That is why it is also known as 'request form' (e.g., Takada and Endo 2015: 53). The data contain a total of 423 such instances – an average of almost 4 per encounter. Only 8 interactions occur without any V-*te* requests, whereas in extreme cases, an encounter may contain up to 15 such cases (on the general problem of counting requests, see Antaki and Kent 2012: 879).

Though perhaps obvious, the overall majority of V-*te* requests are issued by the care workers. As can be understood from Table 6.1, only 36 (8.5%) of all requests of this type are made by a resident. And even though there are numerous other ways of making a control act, as we will see below, these figures illustrate that in most cases, it is the care workers who request something to be done from the residents rather than vice versa.

As mentioned above, V-*te* requests can occur with or without an accompanying *kudasai*. When *kudasai* is omitted, the request is commonly perceived as non-formal in style. An example is *ashi agete* 'Raise your feet' (#21'11) as opposed to *ashi agete kudasai* 'Please raise your feet' (#79'31). It is this non-formal request type that is predominantly used in the data. Table 6.1 shows that it occurs in almost 82% of the cases. This is in line with – and in fact one

Table 6.1 Types of V-*te* requests

	Staff	*Residents*	*Sum*
Non-formal	315 (74.5%)	31 (7.3%)	346 (81.8%)
Formal	72 (17.0%)	5 (1.2%)	77 (18.2%)
Total	**387 (91.5%)**	**36 (8.5%)**	**423 (100%)**

Note: In the non-formal category there occurred one case each of V-*te choodai*, V-*te kure*, V-*te tteba*, V-*teyuno*, and V-*te tte*. In addition, there were 13 instances of the negated form V-*nai de*. Negative requests in the formal style (V-*nai de kudasai*) were not contained.

Table 6.2 Verbs used in V-*te* requests

Verb	Frequency
ageru 'raise'	50 (11.4%)
tsukamaru 'hold tight'	41 (9.7%)
matsu 'wait'	37 (8.7%)
osu 'push'	24 (5.7%)
motsu 'hold'	23 (4.4%)
suwaru 'sit down'	19 (4.5%)
ireru 'insert'	19 (4.5%)
yobu 'call'	16 (3.8%)
nobasu 'stretch'	12 (2.8%)
yorikakaru 'lean on'	10 (4.4%)
Others (n=80)	172 (40.7%)

Note: In auxiliary constructions like V-*te ite*, V-*te oite*, and V-*te shimatte*, the main verb was counted.

contributing factor to – the predominance of non-formal speech in the data overall, as observed in section 4.2.1.

A closer look at the most frequent verbs in V-*te* requests reveals how most of these control acts call for an instant physical action by the care recipient. They qualify for what Vine (2004: 32–33) refers to as 'now requests'. As can be seen in Table 6.2, the list is headed by *ageru*, prototypically used for asking a resident to raise a certain part of their body (hands, head, feet), as in the example just discussed. The second most frequent V-*te* verb is *tsukamaru*, which requests a resident to hold tight to some fixed object, in preparation for a transfer. Other verbs that demand swift physical action vis-à-vis an impending care task are *motsu* 'hold' (e.g., one's own arm while being moved), *suwaru* 'sit down' (e.g., on the toilet after moving over), *ireru* 'insert' (e.g., slipping one's head into a sweater, see excerpt 6.2), *nobasu* 'stretch' (e.g., one's arm while being dressed), and *yorikakaru* 'lean on' (e.g., the care worker).

The list in Table 6.2 contains only three verbs that do not call for the prompt performance of an imminent physical action: *osu* 'push' and *yobu* 'call', both of which in Vine's (2004) terminology qualify as 'later requests' in that they refer to the temporally more remote act of pressing the nurse call after using the toilet (also see section 5.2), and *matsu* 'wait', which requests non-action rather than action. The 37 *matsu* requests fall into two basic types. They either function as announcements of a care worker's temporary leave, or are used in an attempt to prevent or 'brake' undesired resident movements (see also section 7.2).

Apart from V-*te* requests, a second common format for control acts is utterances with verbs in volitional form, which creates a hortative request. The sample contains a total of 162 such cases. The closest corresponding English form would be a construction with 'let's', as in *toire ikoo* (#16'9) or, in formal style, *o-toire ikimashoo* (#35'27), both of which could best be translated as 'Let's go

Table 6.3 Types of hortatives

	Staff	*Residents*	*Sum*
***V-(y)oo* 'Let's'**	105 (64.8%)	2 (1.2%)	107 (66.0%)
Non-formal	51 (31.5%)	2 (1.2%)	53 (32.7%)
Formal	54 (33.3%)		54 (33.3%)
***V-(y)oo ka* 'Shall we'**	50 (30.9%)	5 (3.1%)	55 (34.0%)
Non-formal	33 (20.4%)	4 (2.5%)	37 (22.8%)
Formal	17 (10.5%)	1 (0.6%)	18 (11.1%)
Total	**155 (95.7%)**	**7 (4.3%)**	**162 (100%)**

Note: The copula volitionals *deshoo*(*ka*) and *daroo*(*ka*) were excluded from the analysis since they have various functions that do not qualify as control acts (see McGloin 2002). *V-(y)oo ka* includes two instances without *ka* that were clearly pronounced as interrogatives.

to the toilet'. When the interrogative marker *ka* is attached, the request is transformed into a question. Examples are *o-toire ikooka* (#23'50) and its formal correspondent *o-toire ikimashooka* (#36'22), the most approximate translation of which would be 'Shall we go to the toilet?'

Table 6.3 shows the occurrence of the two hortative forms in the sample. Here, too, and even more so than with V-*te* requests, the overwhelming majority of the utterances are produced by the care workers. Of all 162 instances, a mere seven (4.3%) are contained in utterances by the residents.

The use of 'let's' and first person plural pronouns has been criticised by previous researchers as 'false collaborative' (West 1990: 97) or 'pseudo participation' (Ervin-Tripp 1976: 84, Holmes 1983: 102). Yet while Ryan and her colleagues (1995: 151) explicitly cite 'exclusive and overinclusive *we*' as one component of patronising talk (but also see Wood and Ryan 1991: 180–181), other studies on communication in eldercare evaluate such forms in more favourable ways. For instance, Herzberger classifies inclusive 'we' as a positive politeness strategy intended to reduce the distance between caregiver and care recipient. Likewise, Marsden and Holmes (2014: 22) regard the use of 'let's' as a strategy to present a directive as a 'jointly constructed cooperative action'. Posenau (2014: 69) recognises the use of the German 'nurse *we*' as an acknowledgment of a resident's active participation in an impending task, even where the main physical burden is on the care worker. A similar point has been made by Sachweh, though she explicitly discourages 'we' in the care context as being 'unprofessional and unnecessary' (Sachweh 2005: 116).

The frequent occurrence of hortative forms in the present study raises similar issues. While their use may be motivated to foreground the active role of a resident during the care activities, it certainly does have patronising features (see, e.g., the example sentences in Usami and Endō 1997: 67). On the other hand, it must be acknowledged that requests in hortative format are very common in Japanese everyday life overall (e.g., Wetzel 2010: 325, Backhaus 2016), a point that further complicates attempts at cross-cultural comparison of this type of control act.

While V-*te* requests and hortatives clearly constitute the two most common forms for control acts in the data, there are a huge number of other forms to be found, expressing considerably different degrees of entitlement to a request. On the one end of the scale, there is what Ervin-Tripp (1976: 29) calls 'permission directives', as in the interrogative V-*te moratte ii*? (e.g., LN-*san chotto matte moratte ii desu ka*? 'LN-*san* could you wait (for me) just a second?' #32'109f). The formal style and question format here emphasise the resident's authority to grant permission, whereas the benefactive verb *morau* marks the care worker as the receiver of this permission. In addition, the adverb *chotto* 'a little' is used to downsize the imposition of the requested action (see also Jansson and Plejert 2014: 51).

But control acts can also be formulated in much more straightforward ways. For instance, the data contain a large number of 'announcements' that take a resident's cooperation with a coming action for granted. Examples are *hai ikima:su* 'Okay, here we go' (#41'76) or *tatsu yo:* 'You/we'll stand up now' (#50'66). Another considerably direct way of performing a control act is through noun phrase-based instructions that simply name the object something is required to be done with. The care workers frequently issue directives such as *hai hantai no ashi* 'Okay other foot' (#23'23), FN-*san uwagi* 'FN-*san* jacket' (see excerpt 6.1), or just *te* 'Hand' (#100'98). As we will see in the next chapter, the material mentioned in these phrases is often repeated, in an attempt to speed up the accomplishment of the required action (see section 7.2).

Taking a closer look at control acts in interaction, the data show that they are frequently performed without a subsequent verbal reaction by a resident. An example is presented in excerpt 6.1, in which a care worker is helping a resident out of bed. The passage contains a series of four control acts: a hortative form requesting the resident to bend her knees (line 10), an overall

Excerpt 6.1 (#101'10–17)

10	CW	*hiza, mageyoo*
		Let's bend your knees.
11		(2.8)
12		*okosu yo*
		I'm getting you up now.
13		(1.8)
14		*ashi hirogete,*
		Stretch out your legs.
15		(1.8)
16		FN-*san uwagi*
		FN-*san* your jacket
17		(1.1)

announcement that the care worker will now get her up (line 12), a V-*te* request asking the resident to stretch out her legs (line 14), and a noun phrase instruction consisting of a term of address (in vocative function, see section 4.1) and the object to be worked on – the resident's jacket (line 16).

Given the smooth progress of the sequence, it is safe to assume that each of the required actions (except for the more global 'I'm getting you up now' in line 12) is performed immediately after the respective directive, during the subsequent pauses in lines 11, 15, and 17. In terms of sequential structure, the excerpt thus shows how each control act verbalised by the care worker constitutes a first pair part (FPP), the corresponding second pair part (SPP) of which is produced by the resident not through verbal action, but through 'embodied fulfilment' (Rauniomaa and Keisanen 2012: 831) of the requested physical action. In other words, a control act sequence minimally consists of an adjacency pair with a verbal FPP, followed by an SPP that may be, and in fact commonly is, left non-verbalised.

Excerpt 6.2 presents additional evidence for the pervasiveness of this pattern in task talk. It shows the participants during the dressing, with the care worker providing a number of detailed instructions about what the resident should do next: first, slip in her hand (line 76), then stretch it (line 78), and finally stand up to move back into the wheelchair (line 80). Here, too, the instructions are received (and promptly executed) by the resident without any verbal acknowledgment. The one deviation from the pattern is in line 83, where the resident explicitly confirms the care worker's preceding suggestion that she should get up again at 6 o'clock (after getting back to her room for another brief nap – it is now 4:50). This is the only directive in the excerpt that calls for – and would be hard to respond to without – verbal action. The resident's verbalisation of the SPP at this point shows that she is well aware of the difference between the two types of control acts.

Excerpt 6.2 (#47'76–83)

76	CW	*te ireyoo* Let's slip in your hand.
77		(10.5)
78		*te nobashite:* Stretch out your hand.
79		(2.2)
80		*ii yo tatte* Right, you can stand up.
81		(17.0)
82		*ja:ne, rokuji sugi ni nattara okiyoo ne* Okay then, let's get up when it's past six.
83	Res	*a::* Uh-huh

As the two excerpts exemplify, the default reaction to a control act FPP that calls for a physical action, or, as Antaki and Kent (2012: 887) put it, seeks 'an immediate physical change in the world', is the prompt delivery of that action in SPP position. Most commonly, this is done without any verbal ado, in a very similar way as observed by Korkiakangas et al. (2016) in a study on doctors' control acts to medical staff in the operating theatre. And while the present data sample, like Korkiakangas et al.'s study, does contain examples where a requested action is accompanied by a brief verbal acknowledgment (see, e.g., excerpt 5.12, lines 44–45), these are more the exception than the rule in the setting under observation.

6.1.2 Inquiries

Counter to the care workers' overwhelming predominance in making requests and other control acts, task talk also commonly contains speech acts that explicitly transfer the right to decide about a current or coming action to the residents. The most common type of such speech acts is inquiries by the care workers: Are you ready to move over? Which sweater would you like to wear? Would you like to put on a jacket before we leave? Have you finished using the toilet yet? These are some of the regular issues that require a resident's confirmation in order to proceed with the tasks.

This subsection takes a closer look at the basic structural properties of inquiry sequences. We move right into the data with excerpt 6.3. It presents an exchange between a care worker and a resident during the dressing tasks. The question that arises in this excerpt is if the resident would like to put on a cardigan. This is what the care worker inquires about in line 38, which constitutes the first pair part (FPP) of the newly evolving sequence. The resident replies in the affirmative in line 39, thus providing the corresponding second pair part (SPP). In a final step, the care worker acknowledges the resident's reply with a sequence closing third (SCT).

One regular topic of inquiry is whether a current care task has been (or is about to be) completed, which is a necessary requirement to move on to the next task. An example is given in excerpt 6.4, where we observe the participants as they are working on the resident's shoes. In line 104, the care worker asks the resident if she has her heels in, which is the FPP that opens up the sequence. The resident delivers her affirmative reply in SPP position in the next turn, which is – again – followed by an SCT by the care worker, in line 106. Note

Excerpt 6.3 (#95'38–40)

38	CW	*kimasu ka*
		Are you putting it on?
39	Res	*un,* [*kiru(yo)*
		Uh-huh, I am
40	CW	[*un*
		Uh-huh

Excerpt 6.4 (#10'104–106)

104	CW	*kakato hairimashita?* Have you got your heels in?
105	Res	*hai,* [*hairimashita* Yes, I'm in.
106	CW	[*hai* Okay

Excerpt 6.5 (#83'55–59)

55	CW	*hairimashita ka ne* Have you got in?
56		(1.1)
57		*haitta ka*[*shira* You've got in?
58	Res	[*hai, haitte masu*[, *arigatoo gozaimasu* Yes, I have, thank you
59	CW	[*unn* Uh-huh

that in both this and the previous example, the care worker's SCT is delivered in partial overlap with the resident's preceding SPP, a phenomenon to which we will come back in the next chapter (see section 7.1).

The two excerpts show that inquiry sequences normally take on a minimal structure of three turns: an FPP by the care worker that introduces the topic of the inquiry, an SPP in which the resident provides a (normally affirmative) reply to the inquired topic, and an SCT by the care worker that acknowledges the resident's reply (see also Schegloff 2007: 120–123). Though difficult to quantify, a look through the transcripts reveals that an inquiry sequence is hardly ever left without a sequence closing third by a care worker. Incidentally, the same to some extent applies to other types of sequences, including greeting exchanges, as we have seen in section 5.1 (see excerpt 5.2).

Another property of inquiry sequences is that a resident's reaction to a care worker's FPP may not be delivered right on the spot. In such cases, the care worker often reacts by offering a subsequent version of the pending FPP, which marks the absence of the expected second pair part, in an attempt to speed up its delivery. We have come across a similar case in the analysis of the openings in the previous chapter (see excerpt 5.3). The passage presented in excerpt 6.5 demonstrates that such prodding is a common feature in inquiry sequences, too.

As in excerpt 6.4, the task that is being completed here is putting on a resident's shoes. The care worker with her question in line 55 checks if the resident has slipped them on properly. Not getting a direct reply, she repeats her question in line 57, this time in plain style (*haitta* rather than *hairimashita*) and with a different question marker (*kashira* rather than *ka ne*). The resident, partly in overlap with this second question, in line 58 replies that he has put his shoes on correctly, to which he adds a token of gratitude. As usual, this is acknowledged by the care worker with a sequence closing third in line 59, which marks the end of the inquiry sequence.

The examples presented in this subsection show that, unlike the default format for control acts, an inquiry sequence normally takes a three-tiered, (FPP) (SPP) (SCT) structure. One possible and quite common extension is an additionally inserted turn after the initially delivered FPP in such cases where a resident's SPP is not produced within the time frame the care worker considers appropriate. We will come back to such inserts, which are quite pervasive in the data, in the next chapter (see section 7.3).

6.1.3   Transition marker hai,

A third and in fact most essential component of task talk is the little word *hai* (literally, 'yes'). Previous research has increasingly revealed that *hai* is a highly complex interactional device, which according to sequential context can have a great variety of functions (Hinata 1980, Kitagawa 1980, Angles et al. 2000, Miyake 2001, Togashi 2002, Takagi 2008, Tanaka 2010, Yamamoto 2016). However, it seems that the specific way it is predominantly used in the present data has not been given much attention so far.

This subsection will show that *hai* in resident–staff interactions most commonly works as a task transition marker. Employed in this way, it comes with a rising intonation (*hai,*) and does two things at once: announces the end of a running task and, in so doing, paves the way for the beginning of a new task. This is partially in line with McGloin's (1998: 118) observation that *hai,* is 'highly oriented to making the next move in an interaction'. According to Angles et al. (2000: 62), *hai,* used in this way serves as a 'promoter'. It thus falls into the group of what Bangerter and Clark (2003: 197) refer to as 'navigation tools' that help participants 'move through joint activities'. The closest English approximation for this type of *hai,* would be 'okay' (e.g., Kitagawa 1980: 114), which is how I have translated it in the transcripts most of the time (for an extensive discussion of the various functions of 'okay' in medical settings, see Beach 1995).

As observed by Furuta and Horie (2014), *hai,* as a task transition marker frequently comes together with an announcement of the new task. This creates a control act FPP with *hai,* in turn-initial position. Excerpt 6.6 contains three examples. The interaction takes place after the care worker has accompanied the resident to the toilet. She has just asked the resident to remove her feet from the wheelchair's footrests. In line 66, the care worker's *hai,* acknowledges that this has been done. In the same turn, she also announces the next task, which is to stand up from the wheelchair. What follows is a pause of 2.7 seconds, the approximate time it takes for the resident to do so. Completion of the task is signalled with another *hai,* by the care worker in line 68, again directly followed by a new task announcement: that she will now pull down the resident's trousers. Line 70 follows the same pattern, with *hai,* marking

Excerpt 6.6 (#36'66–71)

66	CW	*hai, ja tachimashoo*
		Okay, let's stand up then
67		(2.7)
68		*hai, zubon sagemasu yo*
		Okay, I pull down your trousers
69		(5.0)
70		*hai, doozo o-kake kudasai*
		Okay, please sit down
71		(0.7)

Excerpt 6.7 (#44'19–30)

19	CW	*hai,*
		Okay
20		(6.5)
21		*hai,*
		Okay
22		(7.5)
23		*hai,*
		Okay
24		(6.0)
25		*hai,*
		Okay
26		(3.5)
27		*hai,*
		Okay
28		(5.0)
29		*hai,*
		Okay
30		(15.0)

the completion of the running task plus an announcement of the new task, having the resident sit down on the toilet seat. Note that, in line with the analysis in section 6.1.1, all three control act FPPs are reacted to by the resident with a non-verbalised performance of the requested action in SPP position (lines 67, 69, 71).

Hai, as a task transition marker can also form a full turn on its own. In extreme cases, this may result in exchanges that consist almost exclusively of *hai,* turns. Excerpt 6.7 is one such example. It starts briefly after the opening, with the resident just having agreed to get up and the care worker now getting her ready for the toilet. Each of the tasks performed between lines 19 and 30 on completion (or so we may assume) is marked by the care worker with *hai,*, followed by a long silence during which a new task is being performed – whose completion is to be announced with another *hai,*, and so forth. The participants here show a closely attuned understanding of the task flow, which works without any further specification through language. The verbal action merely serves to time the tasks, not to name them.

Excerpt 6.7 illustrates how a large number of routine tasks can be performed virtually without any verbal instructions. A single token suffices to mark the completion of a running task and at the same time announce that a new task is on the way. The resulting adjacency pairs of a *hai,* signal (FPP) and a subsequently performed non-verbal action (SPP) can be considered the shortest possible format for a control act sequence in the data.

The importance of task transition markers in care communication has been observed in a number of studies from other cultural contexts. Grainger (1993b: 206) in her data from Wales has identified the common usage of discourse markers such as 'Okay', 'Right', and 'Alright then' to structure an interaction and work through the different care tasks. In German eldercare, a number of one-word tokens fulfil a similar function. As Posenau (2014: 89) observes, these 'framing particles' frequently occur after long silences to announce an upcoming new task (see also Sachweh 2000: 123, 2005: 73), just as we have seen in the two *hai,* excerpts. Similar observations have been made by Engbersen (2009) in a study on communication in a care facility in the Netherlands, where the discourse marker 'nou' was frequently used as a 'verbal articulator of closing a sequence interactionally and physically completing a stage in the course of action'. Though there may be slight differences for each of the forms mentioned, the similarities are quite striking. Future studies may help to explore how universal the phenomenon is in care communication around the globe.

6.1.4 *Heave-hoes*

A final component of task talk that deserves special attention is what for lack of a better term I will refer to as 'heave-hoes'. The Japanese expression for this category of words is *kakegoe.* Even more so than *hai,*, heave-hoes are intimately linked to the performance of some physical action (Udo 2007, Hosoma 2016: 47–52, 59–61). As will be seen, a heave-ho commonly occurs at the onset of such an action or slightly in advance of it. It can be performed by a single person or by two (or more) persons collaborating with an action. In this second case, it also fulfils an important coordinative function.

The most frequent heave-ho in the data is *yoisho,* which is characterised by Fukuda (2005: 1045) as a 'set phrase used when one engages in work that requires physical strength, such as carrying, lifting, and pushing a heavy item'. *Yoisho* occurs in the corpus no less than 252 times. If slightly variant forms such as *iyoisho, issho, sshi, yoisho,* and *yoishotto,* as well as more remote derivatives like *yokkorasho, yokkorase,* and *dokkoisho,* are included, the total number comes to 475. This means that *yoisho* tokens occur more than 4 times on average in each of the 107 morning care interactions. A second heave-ho that is a common complement of task-talk is *se:no* and its variants, including *isse:no/* and *se:no se/.* They occur 62 times in the corpus. Finally, various forms of the counting formula *ichi ni* 'one, two' are used a total of 29 times (see Table 6.4 below).

The main difference between the three types of heave-ho forms is their timing with respect to the action they accompany. Their occurrence in the data suggests that *se:no* and *ichi ni* are used to prepare an immediately impending action. *Yoisho,* on the other hand, is delivered during the very performance of that action. In other words, *se:no* and *ichi ni* can be conceived of as a 'Ready?' signal, to which *yoisho* provides the corresponding 'Go!' The two types of heave-hoes thus can, and frequently do, occur in sequence, verbalising the preparation of an action with *se:no* or *ichi ni*, and the performance itself with *yoisho*. A similar phenomenon has been identified by Posenau (2014: 95–96) in his German data, where the counting formula 'eins, zwei' was combined with the 'Go' signal 'hoppala'.

Excerpt 6.8 exemplifies three different uses of heave-hoes from one interaction. The first sequence (lines 92–99) shows how care worker and resident each

Excerpt 6.8 (#13'92–99, 160–165, 194–197)

92	CW	*hai*, FN-*san atama ireru yo* Okay, FN-san I insert your head now
93	Res	*nn* Uh-huh
94		(0.7)
95	CW	*iyoisho* ((heave-ho))
96		(1.0)
97		*hai, migi te* Okay, right hand
98		(2.0)
99	Res	*yoisho* ((heave-ho))
((61 lines skipped))		
160	CW	*hai,* [*tatsu yo* Okay, (we/you) stand up
161	Res	[*uhunnnhhun* ((grunting))
162	CW	*se::no::se/* ((heave-ho))
163		(1.5)
164		[*hai* Okay
165	Res	[*yoisho* ((heave-ho))
((29 lines skipped, moving to toilet))		
194	CW	*hai,* (0.3) *iku yo*:= Okay, here we go
195	Res	=*unn*= Uh-huh
196	CW	=*se:no:/ iyo*= ((heave-ho)) ((heave-))
197	Res	=*yoisho* ((heave-ho))

deliver one heave-ho 'for themselves', that is, separately and during different actions. The care worker's *(i)yoisho* in line 95 occurs while she is pulling a sweater or some other piece of clothing over the resident's head. The resident delivers her *yoisho* several seconds later (line 99), after the care worker has asked her to produce her right hand, most likely in order to pull the resident's arm through the same piece of clothing.

The next sequence (lines 160–165) is from a part of the interaction where the resident transfers from bed to wheelchair. This is announced as the next task by the care worker in line 160 (in part overlapping with the resident's continuous grunting, which occurs throughout the exchange). In order to properly time the action of standing up, which requires some non-trivial degree of cooperation from the resident, the care worker in line 162 uses *se::no::se/* as a 'Ready?' signal. The next audible action is a precise overlapping of the care worker's *hai* with the resident's *yoisho* heave-ho (lines 164–165). We can be sure that this marks the point where the physical action is performed.

The task in the third sequence (lines 194–197) is making the resident stand up from the wheelchair in order to have her move over to the toilet. The care worker announces this in line 194 and it is acknowledged by the resident in line 195. Just like in the previous sequence, the care worker then uses *se:no:/* to prepare the resident for the directly impending action. The start of the action itself can be heard coinciding with the care worker's *iyo*, a variant form of *yoisho*, at the end of line 196. With some minimal delay, the resident responds with a *yoisho* heave-ho on her part (line 197), latched to the care worker's previous turn. In contrast to the second sequence, this suggests that the two participants' actions here do not entirely coincide but happen in direct succession. They are as 'latched' to each other as their verbalisations.

The three examples show that *yoisho* can be used in two structurally different ways. In the first sequence (lines 92–99), as in the majority of the cases in the data, it occurs as a single, self-sufficient turn that is produced by one of the participants during the performance of some physical action. In these cases, it is frequently delivered with a low voice, closely resembling soliloquy. In the second (lines 160–165) and third sequences (lines 194–197), *yoisho* functions as a second pair part (SPP) of an adjacency pair whose first pair part (FPP) is a *se:no* heave-ho. Special about this adjacency pair is that it does not necessarily involve speaker change. As the second and third sequences show, the care worker delivers both FPP and SPP (in the former case, *hai*, rather than *yoisho*) by herself, thus creating an overlap (second sequence) or latching (third sequence) with the resident's concurring SPP.

One noteworthy point here is that *yoisho* as SPP is commonly delivered by both participants (almost) simultaneously, thus suspending a fundamental rule of the turn-taking system: one party at a time (Sacks et al. 1974). When *se:no* or a similar item is used as FPP to prepare for an imminent action, the following SPP – *yoisho* or other – is not only allowed but expected to be delivered by all participants involved in that action (for other examples of such 'choral' forms of talk, see Schegloff 2000: 6). The result is the observed overlap (lines 164–165) or latching (lines 196–197) of turns. The reason why there is a complete overlap in the second

Table 6.4 Occurrence and staff/resident ratio of heave hoes

Type of heave-ho	Care workers	Residents	Total
yoisho	419 (88%)	56 (12%)	475 (100%)
se:no	60 (97%)	2 (3%)	62 (100%)
ichi ni	24 (83%)	5 (17%)	29 (100%)

Note: All three heave-ho types include variant forms with slightly different phonetic realisations.

sequence, as opposed to a mere near-overlap in the third one, appears to arise from the different ways in which the two actions are performed. The overlap in the second sequence suggests that the resident's and the care worker's movements are precisely synchronised, whereas in the third sequence, the care worker seems to initiate a movement that is taken over by the resident just one instance later.

Quantitatively speaking, the overall majority of all heave-hoes are delivered by the care workers. As shown in Table 6.4, 88% of all *yoisho* forms, 97% of the *se:no* tokens, and 83% of the *ichi ni* counts are contained in turns by the care workers. This, again, and in a quite literal sense, reveals the care workers' dominating role in driving the action along.

On a critical note, it has to be acknowledged that the 'invisibility' of the data must leave any closer examination of heave-hoes in the sample somewhat speculative. As video data are not available, the action line has to be reconstructed from the audio information, including previous announcements of an action by one of the participants, prosodic features of the heave-ho in question, and cues from the background noise. This involves some risk of circularity in that the verbal output is taken as a result and thus 'proof' of an action whose actual performance cannot be definitely confirmed except by the verbal output itself. It is obvious that for more detailed research on heave-hoes and other action-related utterance types, video data are indispensable.

6.1.5 Silence

One final characteristic to note in the context of task talk is the very absence of such talk, and in fact, of any talk at all. As can be seen in Table 6.5, long stretches of silence are a common feature of the morning care exchanges. The transcripts contain a total of 482 pauses between 5 and 10 seconds, 444 pauses between 10 and 60 seconds, and 12 pauses in which the participants work in silence for even longer than that. The most extensive silence of the sample is a pause of no less than 83 seconds, which occurs while a care worker is dressing a resident before they move over to the toilet (#96).

Excerpt 6.9 exemplifies how a minimal degree of talk can suffice to handle all necessary activities of the morning care. The unabridged transcript has 21 lines but only 8 of these contain recognisable verbal material, mostly from the care worker and virtually none from the resident (who does not suffer from

Table 6.5 Pauses longer than 5 seconds

Pause length	Frequency
5–9 secs	482
10–19 secs	304
20–29 secs	86
30–39 secs	28
40–49 secs	18
50–59 secs	8
60+ secs	12

Note: Does not include pauses during which the participants were temporarily physically separated and/or talked to someone else than each other.

Excerpt 6.9 (#6'1–21)

1	CW	((enters room))
2		(9.0, opens bed curtains, other preparations)
3		*ohayo:* Morning
4		(0.2)
5	Res	*nn:go:* ((reply to greeting))
6		(12.5)
7		((grunts/snorts))
8		(46.5)
9	CW	*hai,* Okay
10		(7.0)
11		*hai,* Okay
12		(23.3, to toilet)
13		*tatsu yo:* (We/you) stand up
14		(2.7)
15		*se:no, iennfu* ((heave-ho)) ((heave-ho))
16		(23.5)
17		*owattara oshite ne* When you've finished push
18		(1.1)
19		*owattara oshite ne* When you've finished push
20		(1.8)
21		((leaves))

any type of aphasia – we hear him speak in several other exchanges – though he has some obvious problems with articulation).

After the opening phase, consisting of the usual preparations (lines 1–2) and a greeting adjacency pair with a somewhat unclearly pronounced second pair part (line 3–5), the interaction moves directly into the main part. The participants work through the tasks mostly in silence, except for a one-time grunting or snorting by the resident (line 7) and a few of the common task talk elements by the care worker: two occurrences of *hai,* (lines 9 and 11) during activities in the resident's room, and a directive announcement to stand up (line 13) when at the toilet, followed by a heave-ho interjection while the action is performed (line 15). The interaction closes with two reminders by the care worker to call when finished (lines 17 and 19), which constitutes the terminal exchange of the encounter.

The quantification in Table 6.6 shows that interactions like the one just described are quite common. Excluding greetings and similar phatic elements from the openings and closings, at least 39 of the 107 morning care exchanges do not contain any non-task related talk at all. And just like in excerpt 6.9, most of these interactions are dominated by longer stretches of silence, interspersed with brief instances of task talk only where it becomes necessary to verbally coordinate an activity. These findings are in line with Grainger's (2004b, see 2.2.) observation that absence of talk and task-oriented talk are two general characteristics of care communication.

6.2   Non-task talk

Despite the predominance of task talk, the data presented in Table 6.6 also show that the residents and the care workers in Edogawa Care do have something else than task-related matters to tell each other when they get together

Table 6.6 Occurrence of non-task talk sequences per interaction

Non-task talk sequences per interaction	*Number of interactions*
0	39 (36.4%)
1	26 (24.3%)
2	17 (15.9%)
3	11 (10.3%)
4	7 (6.5%)
5	2 (1.9%)
6	4 (3.7%)
8	1 (0.9%)
Total	**107 (100%)**

in these early hours of the day. This section takes a closer look at what exactly that is, how it is brought up, and by whom.

6.2.1   *Topics*

As defined in the introductory part to this chapter, non-task talk includes all instances of talk that do not directly relate to the running care tasks. In total, the data contain 163 such sequences. Table 6.7 shows that the most frequent topic is the previous night, discussed in 24 of the interactions. Normally initiated by some sort of 'Did you sleep well?' question by the care worker, sequences of this type tend to occur soon after the beginning of an interaction – which is why in some studies they are considered part of the opening (e.g., Posenau 2014: 83) – and do not develop into longer exchanges. We have discussed two examples in section 4.2 (see excerpts 4.2 and 4.3).

A second major topic is other residents, such as the roommate lying in bed with her shoes on (#89) or the person crying in the room next door (#59). In quite a few cases, a resident comments on, or is informed about, how many other residents are already up (#19, #32, #73, #77, #82). While the majority of these sequences are relatively short, the data also contain a few longer exchanges. In one such case, a male resident is teasing a male care worker about his being adored by a female resident from the same floor, a topic that continues through over 80 consecutive lines (#59). Another example is a female

Table 6.7 Topics discussed in non-task talk

Topics	Number of times raised
Last night	24
Other residents	20
Today's events	14
Outside	13
Time	13
Resident's home/family	11
Resident's things	10
Staff shifts	10
Research/Researchers	10
Resident's constitution	9
Joking/verbal play	7
Care worker's constitution	5
Others	17
Sum	**163**

Note: Sequences reinitiating a previously raised topic were counted separately.

resident's complaint about her lecherous male peers who keep trying to peek through her clothes (#66, see section 6.3).

The 14 sequences about 'Today's events' mainly deal with the topic of bathing, a very important part of Japanese everyday life (Clark 1992), and life in Edogawa Care, too. As described in section 3.1, each floor has a large community bathing space used by all residents two days a week. On Mondays, the male residents are the first to use the bathing space, right after breakfast, whereas on Thursdays, the women go first. The individual order within the two groups of residents changes each bathing day. It is determined by number cards distributed to the residents during the previous night. Hence, 'What is your number today?' is a topic discussed at some length in three of the interactions (#35, #84, #92), while in others, plans for the day are made with explicit reference to the bathing (e.g., #61). The topic occasionally becomes raised even on non-bathing days, such as in a brief sequence in which a care worker observes that today is not a bathing day (#33). A second regular institutional 'event' is today's change of sheets, which is discussed in three of the interactions (#51, #53, #100).

In total, the data contain only two sequences that deal with coming events not immediately part of the daily institutional routine. Both occur in a conversation between a female care worker and a male resident scheduled for an outpatient exam, after which his son will take him home for the day (#83). Parts of this rather exceptional sequence have been discussed in section 4.3 (see excerpt 4.6). The fact that the routinised events of the institution provide the main source for conversations about the day suggests that there is not much else expected to happen that would be worth talking about in Edogawa Care, or at least not during the morning care activities.

The topic area 'Outside' comprises two main types of contents. One is the weather, real (#70) or as forecasted (#33), which is one of the most prototypical topics for small talk, not only in Japan (see Coupland and Ylänne-McEwen 2000). The second is the coming of daybreak, frequently referred to in comments such as 'It's still pitch-dark outside' (#59). A related topic is the time, which in most cases is brought up at a relatively early stage of an interaction, either by way of a resident's inquiry (#3) or announced by a care worker (#16). As we have seen in section 5.1.2, time is a frequent component in negotiations about getting up.

Various groups of topics are closely related to the residents, their belongings, physical constitution, and family or pre-institutional life. In one sequence, a care worker wants to know about yesterday's visit by a resident's wife (#9); in another one, a resident complains about frequently being scolded by her daughter for being overweight (#10). In contrast to these relatively short exchanges, there are longer sequences in which residents talk about their earlier life. One resident particularly eager to raise such topics is Rm093, whom we have met in chapter 4 when discussing his somewhat extraordinary choice of address terms (see excerpt 4.1). He discloses to the care workers such intimate issues as his infertility (#73) and his misbehaviour when he was young (#82), among others.

Though the group of care workers becomes a topic of non-task talk far less frequently, they are not entirely exempt from being talked about. A frequent topic of inquiry by the residents is the duty roster, addressed with questions such as 'When is your next night shift?' (#82) or 'Who will be on today's day shift?' (#73). In one case, a resident compliments the care worker by stating that she is very happy that 'it's you who's waking me up today'. The care worker does her best to play down this compliment, laughingly pointing out that all staff members do their job 'just the same' (#84). Cases in which a care worker's non-institutional background becomes a topic of discussion are rare, but occasionally occur, too (see section 6.3).

A related non-task topic is the care workers' physical constitution. Though this category contains only five cases, they deserve special attention as instances of blurred boundaries between carer and cared-for. In two cases, a care worker's complaint about being tired entails various concerned questions and comments by her conversational partner (#43, #97). In two other cases, residents comment on the surgical mask a care worker is wearing that day. This leads her to describe in some detail the cold she has caught (#37, #40, see excerpt 6.15).

As described in section 2.2, previous researchers have stressed the favourable influence of joking and verbal play in care communication (e.g., Lyman 1988, Heinemann 2009a, Marsden and Holmes 2014). My data contain at least seven instances that qualify for this type of non-task talk. One example is a brief sequence in which a care worker jokingly bids a resident goodnight, as though putting her to bed rather than getting her up (#60). Another joking sequence develops from a resident's slip of the tongue, saying *reiboo* 'air conditioner' instead of *danboo* 'heating' (#37). Some instances include verbal play on onomatopoetic expressions and demonstratives (#37, #31). In two other cases, the participants play around with the hyper-formal copula verb *gozaimasu* and its (fake) derivatives *gozansu* and *gojaru* (#37, #89). We have discussed one such instance of honorific role language in section 4.3 (see excerpt 4.8).

A last topic to be mentioned is the two researchers. While my colleague and I were busy trying to keep track of what was going on during recording time, we tended to forget that we were not only being observers but also being observed. Only after we had started the transcribing did we realise that we showed up as a topic in a number of conversations – ten in total. We normally 'occurred' when the resident and the care worker saw us as they were moving through the hallway towards the toilet or the dayroom (e.g., #88), but sometimes were also mentioned without being in sight (e.g., #61). Observer's interference notwithstanding, we were happy that we could provide an additional topic that the people in Edogawa Care would find worthy of talking about.

6.2.2   *Initiating non-task talk*

Having briefly described what types of topics occur during the morning care activities, a next question is who brings up these topics. A quantitative analysis of the 163 non-task talk sequences shows that residents and care workers take on this role to an almost equal extent: 86 (53%) of the sequences are launched by the residents; 77 (47%) by the staff. However, as becomes obvious in Table 6.8, there are some clear preferences with regard to the type of topic.

Table 6.8 Choices of non-task topics

Topics	Introduced by	
	Res.	*Staff*
Last night	7	17
Other residents	14	6
Today's events	3	11
Outside	7	6
Time	10	3
Resident's home/family	7	4
Resident's things	3	7
Staff shifts	10	0
Research/Researchers	8	2
Resident's constitution	1	8
Joking/verbal play	2	5
Care worker's constitution	3	2
Others	11	6
	86	77

Some are prototypical staff topics. These include the previous night and the events for today, clothes and other things belonging to a resident, and her or his constitution. The care workers take a chief interest in institutional matters, particularly the wellbeing of the residents. As care professionals, the morning care to them fulfils an important by-function as a source of gathering information about the residents and their health. By contrast, favourable topics of the residents are their peer residents, the researchers, and the staff shifts. Particularly striking is the distribution of this last topic, which in all ten cases is initiated by the residents, suggesting that the care workers themselves do not like to raise such issues from the other side of the institutional divide.

Perhaps in part owing to these disparate preferences, not all initiations of a non-task topic are equally successful, and it may well happen that one of the participants' explicit attempts to raise a non-task topic will remain unreciprocated by the other. Two such examples are presented below: the first one with a failed attempt by the care worker to initiate a sequence of non-task talk, and the second with reversed roles.

Excerpt 6.10 starts briefly after the opening phase, with the care worker's hortative announcement that she will now get the resident out of bed (line 28). Since the subsequent activities do not require any verbal instructions, the care worker uses this slot to introduce a topic not directly related to the task: that today is bathing day. She makes three consecutive attempts to elicit a reaction from the resident, in lines 30, 32, and 34. Note that each repeat is shorter than the previous one, a phenomenon to be more closely examined

Excerpt 6.10 (#36'28–36)

28	CW	*ja, LN-san okimashoo* Okay, LN-san, let's get up
29		(8.0, CW opens curtains)
30		*kyoo wa o-furo desu yo,* Today is bathing
31		(1.4)
32		*kyoo wa o-furo no hi* Today's bathing day
33		(3.0)
34		*o-furo ne, un* Bathing, you know, uh-huh
35		(5.0)
36		*yoisho* ((heave-ho))

Excerpt 6.11 (#73'159–167)

159	CW	*hai,* Okay
160		(11.0, sound of footsteps from the hallway)
161	Res	*goji kara okita na* He must be up since five
162	CW	*u[n* Uh-huh
163	Res	[*aruiteru yo:* He's walking
164		(0.9)
165		*tontonton tte* 'tap tap tap' he goes
166		(25.0)
167	CW	*hai, dekita* Okay, that's it

in the next chapter (see section 7.3). Yet despite these subsequent versions, the resident, who does not suffer from any speech impairments, does not provide a recognisable verbal response. As a result, the interaction falls silent again until the care worker delivers another task talk item, the heave-ho *yoisho*, in line 36. No further attempt is made to produce any non-task talk after this point.

Initiations of non-task talk sequences may also fail on account of insufficient cooperation by the care worker. Such is the case in excerpt 6.11. The resident is already out of bed and now being dressed. In line 159, the care worker announces the completion of some part of the dressing with transition marker *hai,*. This is followed by 11 seconds during which a new task proceeds without any accompanying talk. At the same time, the sound of footsteps from the hallway becomes audible, indicating that the second care worker is back from the nap room after a brief time-out. Apparently well informed about the break times of the care workers, the resident here initiates a non-task talk sequence about the second care worker being up again (line 161). This is minimally acknowledged by the (first) care worker in line 162, but she is obviously not willing to pursue the topic any further than that. This can be understood from her missing responses to the resident's two follow-ups on the topic in lines 163 and 165. A long silence follows, not to be broken before the next task completion is announced in line 167.

Communication is a cooperative endeavour. As has been obvious in the two examples just discussed, a non-task topic sequence will not make it beyond the first few turns if one of the participants refuses to join in. As to the reasons for the refusal, excerpt 6.11 concurs with the quantitative part of the analysis in showing that the care workers clearly disfavour topics about internal work procedures. The residents on their part can and do reject initiations of non-task talk, too. In the example presented in excerpt 6.10, it seems that the resident simply does not consider the care worker's news that today is a bathing day all that newsworthy. Maybe she found it too trivial, or – who could blame her? – was just not in the mood for a chat after being woken up only a few moments before. Whatever her reasons, we should not forget that different people have different preferences when it comes to talking for the sake of talk itself.

6.3   Shifts

In line with previous studies, one feature of non-task talk sequences is that they are at constant risk of being overruled by an upcoming task that needs to be communicated. As a result, it regularly happens that a running sequence of non-task talk is suspended in order to make room for more 'urgent' matters, and will have to be reactivated once these have been settled. This can entail a large number of shifts back and forth between task and non-task talk, which are the topic of this section.

6.3.1   *In and out of task*

Table 6.9 presents the topic flow of an interaction between a male care worker and a female resident. The exchange as a whole is somewhat out of the ordinary in that the two participants during their 12-minute encounter discuss no less than 6 non-task topics, amounting to a transcript of 600 lines. However, their non-task talk frequently has to compete with shorter inroads of task talk. As the sketch in Table 6.9 shows, each of the non-task talk sequences is suspended by task talk at least once.

Table 6.9 Task and non-task talk in #66

Non-task topic	Sequence	
Resident's compression socks	initiated	by Res
	suspended	by Res
Sewing/Care worker's experiences at vocational college	initiated	by CW
	suspended	by Res
	re-launched	by CW (see excerpt 6.14)
	suspended	by Res (see excerpt 6.14)
	re-launched	by CW (see excerpt 6.14)
	suspended	by Res (see excerpt 6.14)
	re-launched	by CW (see excerpt 6.14)
Sewing machines	initiated	by Res
	suspended	by CW
	failed re-launch	by Res
	re-launched	by CW
Resident's accident with sewing machine	initiated	by Res
	suspended	by CW
	re-launched	by Res
	suspended	by CW (see excerpt 6.12)
	re-launched	by Res (see excerpt 6.12)
	suspended	by CW (see excerpt 6.13)
	failed re-launch	by CW (see excerpt 6.13)
	re-launched	by Res (see excerpt 6.13)
	suspended	by CW
Resident's clothes	initiated	by Res
	suspended	by Res
Other resident	failed initiation	by CW
	initiated	by CW
	suspended	by Res

The first non-task talk sequence arises from a comment by the resident about her compression socks. She finds the socks she has just been given uncomfortable and wonders when her old ones will be back from repair. The second sequence of non-task talk evolves only a few turns later, when a button of the resident's trousers comes off. This is reminiscent of Onoda's (2014, see section 2.3) observation that physical objects are easily turned into conversational objects. In the present case, the care worker apologises for not being able to fix the button, explaining that he cannot sew. This for him provides the starting point to tell a story about his surprise when he went to vocational college and realised that all of his (much younger) classmates had learned to sew at high school.

From this, the talk turns to sewing machines, present and past, which paves the way for a longer story by the resident about an accident she once had with a heavy, old-type sewing machine that was dropped on her foot by 'an idiot' (*baka*) repair service clerk. In the later part of the interaction, the topic returns to the resident's clothes and her worries about being peeked at by lecherous (*sukebe*) male residents. The final topic arises from an incoming nurse call, which

Excerpt 6.12 (#66'314–333)

314	Res	*sore o ko/ kono ashi ni=*
		On this foot
315	CW	*=acha::=*
		Ugh!
316	Res	*=okot(tano),*
		it fell
317		(0.8)
318		*chi darake*
		Blood all over
319	CW	*ara,*
		Oh my
320		(0.5)
321		*itsu itsu kurai no hanashi, sore*
		From about when, when is this story?
322	Res	*wakai* [*toki, uun*
		When I was young
323	CW	[*wakai koro desho, uun, soo da yo ne*
		When you were young, of course.
324		(0.6)
325		*hai, moo ikkai onegai shi* [*ma:su*
		Okay, once more please
326	Res	[*hai, ichi ni: no*
		Okay, one, two,
327		(0.8)
328		[*yoisho*
		((heave-ho))
329	CW	[*yoisho*
		((heave-ho))
330		(1.0)
331	Res	*ta* [*ihen datta yo itakutte*
		It was really awful, painful
332	CW	[*he::,*
		Dear me!
333		*soo da ne, a/, soo da, are omotain da mon ne*
		I see, right, these are heavy, aren't they?

provides an occasion for the care worker to briefly talk about the resident who has just called.

In order to get a better understanding of the mechanism of shifts between task talk and non-task talk, we will take a close-up look at three excerpts from this interaction. The first one, excerpt 6.12, starts when the resident is right in the middle of her story about how the sewing machine came down on her foot. The care worker's use of non-standard response tokens such as *acha::* (line 315) and *ara,* (line 319) displays his emotional involvement as a recipient of the 'scary story' (Sugita 2012) at this point. After the resident has finished her account of the accident, the care worker in line 321 asks when this happened, thus providing a follow-up on the running topic that signalises his interest in the story. The question is answered by the resident somewhat vaguely with 'when I was young', which is taken up and completed by the care worker with a sequence closing third in line 323.

The suspension of the non-task talk sequence occurs in line 325, with the care worker's use of task transition marker *hai*, in turn-initial position, to signalise that the current task has just been finished and a new one is coming up. His attached directive 'once more please' is not intended as a request to the resident to retell her story, obviously, but to cooperate with this next task. That this is directly understood by the resident here, even without any verbal reference to a 'multiactivity moment' (Haddington et al. 2014b: 6), can be seen from her initiation of a heave-ho sequence in line 326, starting while the care worker is still making his request. This prepares the two participants for a very well synchronised, completely overlapping *yoisho* pair in lines 328 and 329.

Once this has been done, the participants swiftly return to the resident's suspended story. This happens almost simultaneously, with a follow-up comment by the resident that 'it [the accident] was really awful' (line 331) and another response token delivered by the care worker virtually at the same time (line 332). The overlap of these two lines demonstrates two characteristics of re-initiating a suspended non-task talk sequence: first, that there may be coordination problems with regard to speaker selection, and second, that both participants share a highly precise understanding about the appropriate timing for getting back from task talk to non-task talk, which is why the overlap occurs in the first place. Of further note is that both participants resume their previous roles as story teller and story recipient, respectively.

While the data contain many other instances of equally well-timed shifts between the two modes of talk, things do not always go as smoothly as in the example just discussed. This can best be understood by taking a closer look at how the interaction continues. The sequel is presented in excerpt 6.13, starting with the last line of excerpt 6.12.

At the beginning of the excerpt, the participants are back at their non-task talk about the resident's accident with the sewing machine. After the care worker has displayed his empathy about the severity of the accident in line 333, the resident continues talking about the state of affairs immediately after the machine hit her foot. While she is still in the middle of her lively account, describing the pain (line 334), her crying, and the 'blood all over' (line 336), the care worker is already back to task. Note that his suspension of the non-task talk sequence is foreshadowed by a would-be soliloquy that some item needs to be the 'other way round' (line 335). This makes the new task 'take a verbal form' (Keisanen et al. 2014: 124), which continues with the care worker's question to the resident if she could 'move this way over there' (line 337). The shift back to task talk is completed in line 338, where the resident replies to the care

333	CW	*soo da ne, a/, soo da, are omotain da mon ne* I see, right, these are heavy, aren't they?
334	Res	*un, omo/ omote ni dete sa*[:, *amari no itasa ni sa=* Uh-huh, I went outside because it was so painful
335	CW	[*hantai nan da* ((to himself)) Other way round
336	Res	=*naki nagara* [*chidarake da kara sa* I was crying, blood all over
337	CW	[*sono mama kotchi ikemasu?* Can you move this way over there?
338	Res	*koo?* Like this?
((20 lines skipped))		
358	Res	*te* Hand
359		(0.5)
360	CW	*un yaru, ashi mo ne=* Uh-huh, I will, and also your feet
361	Res	=*un* Uh-huh
362		(5.0, sound of a zipper)
363	CW	*mishin tsukatta koto nai kara sa:* Because I've never used a sewing machine, you know
364		(0.5)
365	Res	*sorede mishin sa okotta desho* And so it fell down, as I said
366	CW	*un* Uh-huh
367	Res	*dakara sa:,* and that's why
368		(1.2)
369		*mattaku sa:,* really
370		(1.4)
371		*sore de kega shite sa:,* that's how I got injured
372		(0.4)
373		*are dakara sa:,* and that's why
374		(1.2)
375		*uttaete yaru* [*tte* 'I'll sue you for this'
376	CW	[(((laughs))
377	Res	*omotta wake* is what I thought
378	CW	*un* Uh-huh

worker's request with a follow-up question. However, it has taken four full lines with task and non-task talk running parallel to achieve this.

The larger part of the newly evolved task talk sequence has been skipped in the excerpt. Lines 358 to 361 present the closing of the sequence. Note, incidentally, that this is one of the rare cases where a control act is done by a resident (line 358). What follows is a pause of five seconds during which the task continues in silence (only the sound of a zipper being opened or closed is audible). The first one to speak after this is the care worker (line 363) with a re-initiation of the second to last non-task topic: his not knowing how to sew. However, despite his use of the discourse particle *sa:*, which calls for no more than a minimal degree of backchannelling (Morita 2005: 197–198), the resident now launches her own re-initiation of the non-task talk sequence: her story about the accident (line 365). In so doing, she completely ignores both the topical and sequential relevance of the care worker's previous utterance.

Noteworthy about the resident's re-initiation is the opening conjunction *sorede* 'then', here intended to refer back some 30 lines to where the non-task talk sequence was last suspended. Since her story was not finished at this point, she now expresses her entitlement to continue before any other non-task talk may be started or re-activated.

The care worker, on the other hand, who did not seem to expect a follow-up on the resident's story after his previous utterance, now turns into a somewhat less cooperative story recipient than he has been so far. After line 366, he refrains from delivering any more backchannel tokens, despite the resident's continuous calls for these with *sa:* at the end of virtually every line of her multi-turn unit (lines 367–377). The care worker officially resumes his role as story recipient only in line 376, with laughter in response to an unexpected narrative twist in the resident's story. The first standard backchannel token is *un* in line 378, after which the resident is able to finish her story without any more hitches.

As this example shows, the sudden suspension of a non-task talk sequence may entail coordination problems, particularly when the following task talk drags on for some time. In such cases, the participants' understanding about the timing and the appropriateness of re-entry into the pending non-task talk may get out of sync. In the present example, the main problem seems to arise from the fact that the care worker considers the resident's previous story to be largely finished by the time of suspension and hence not really in need of re-initiation, whereas the resident does not.

6.3.2 *Task talk insert by resident*

An interesting point about the discussed exchange as a whole is that it is not necessarily the care worker who suspends non-task talk initiated by the resident, as in the two previous examples, but that it may just be the other way round. As can be seen in Table 6.9, there are quite a number of cases where this happens. Two of them are presented in excerpt 6.14, where the care worker for the first time talks about his experiences at vocational college, while he is helping the

Excerpt 6.14 (#66'151–185)

151	CW	*are desu tte yo,* You know what,
152		(1.0)
153		*ano:* well,
154		(0.5)
155	Res	*chotto mattenno, burajaa ga hazureta* Hang on, my bra has come loose
156		(1.8)
157	CW	*nan dakke* What was I going to say?
158	Res	*nani?* What?
159	CW	*senmon gakkoo ni itteta toki ni ne,* When I went to vocational college,
160	Res	*un,* Uh-huh
161		(0.5)
162	CW	*moo, toshi ga sa:* I was already, you know
163		(0.6)
164	Res	*un* Uh-huh
165		(0.6)
166	CW	*gurutto eto ga isshuu suru kurai=* a whole turn of the zodiac
167		*=hanareterun dake do sa* ahead, you know
168		(0.4)
169		*boku to senmon gakkoosei tte* compared to the other students
170	Res	*ee, ee=* Uh, uh
171	CW	*=un, [de sa:* Uh-huh, and then
172	Res	[*are, kore de ii no ka na?* Wait, is this okay this way?
173	CW	*iin deshoo* Sure it is
174		(0.6)
175		*de,* And
176		(0.9)
177		*sono* these

178		(3.0)
179	Res	*kotchi ka, a[re?* It's here, oh what's that?
180	CW	[*kora ni kiitara* kids when I asked them
181	Res	*un,* Uh-huh
182	CW	*koogyoo kookoo no ko de mo, otoko ga* they said even the boys at the technical high school
183	Res	*un,* Uh-huh
184	CW	*kookoo de, kateika ga atta tte iun da yo* they'd had a home economics class
185	Res	*hE:::* Really?

resident get dressed. He prepares his non-task talk with some sort of 'pre-telling' (Stivers 2013: 193–194) in line 151 and the discourse marker *ano:* in line 153, which signalises that he is claiming the floor for a task non-related story. Just at this point, the resident urgently needs to insert a piece of task talk: that her bra has come loose and needs to be fixed before they can continue the dressing (line 155).

After this task talk interruption, the care worker needs to restart his story (line 157), this time explicitly acknowledged with a 'go ahead' by the resident (line 158), after which the story can finally begin. It unfolds without turbulences through the next couple of turns, in which the care worker tells the resident about the age difference between him and his much younger classmates at college. Noteworthy about this passage are the large gaps that open up between the care worker's utterances and the resident's response tokens (lines 160–166). The verbal interaction seems to be somewhat slowed down here, as the participants need to divert a part of their attention on the 'basso continuo' (Nishizaka 2014: 103) of the task work.

The task becomes verbalised once again in line 172, where the resident has to interrupt the care worker's story a second time. In a slightly soliloquy-like insertion, she wonders whether some (audio-wise irretrievable) part of the presently performed task is 'okay this way'. Note that, as in excerpt 6.13 (line 335), a soliloquy serves as a starting point for the task talk to get a foot in the door. Such types of 'asides' may be a favourable format for shifts back to a task, due to their capacity to communicate a problem with the running task work while at the same time signalising utmost (though necessarily futile) willingness not to interfere with the other's non-task talk.

The care worker responds with a rather brusque confirmation in line 173, before trying to get on with his story in line 175. Here, too, long pauses opening up in his speech suggest a focused concentration on the physical tasks by both participants. Task and non-task talk compete for two more lines, with the resident's verbalisation of some remaining problem with the dressing (line 179), slightly overlapped by the care worker's continuation of his story (line 180). After that, the resident quickly switches back to her role as a story recipient, and the story can go on.

The main point the care worker wants to make in this story, which is going to continue for some 40 more lines, is that unlike his younger classmates, he was never taught how to sew. Telling the story the way he does, he gives away quite a number of personal details about himself, including his age, education, and continuing inability to sew. Of particular note is the fact that the care worker becomes so absorbed in his story that the resident has to call him 'back to task' several times.

6.3.3   *Changing the footing*

The phenomenon of shifting between task talk and non-task talk relates to another noteworthy feature of care communication, which I have elsewhere referred to as institutional role play (see Backhaus 2011). When the participants talk about things unrelated to the care activities, they do not just change the topic, but also change their 'footing'. According to Goffman (1981: 126), this entails 'an alteration in the social capacities in which the persons present claim to be active'.

In the care context, Grainger (1993b: 254) has observed that such instances of 'personal discourse' are 'principally non-institutional and solidary', thus 'allowing the participants to background their institutionally prescribed roles of "nurse" and "patient" and to acknowledge each other as individuals'. Likewise, Posenau (2014: 119) observes that the occurrence of 'care-remote topics' in his German data aims at producing some sort of 'family-like setting, or at least one between persons of equal standing'. Sequences of personal self-disclosure can play an important part in such role shifts, as Heinemann (2007) has shown.

We have already come across similar changes of footing in the previous chapters. For example, in the passage presented in chapter 4 (see excerpt 4.1), the resident's way of addressing the care worker by her first name, in combination with his (somewhat ostentatious) display of considerateness for the 'poor girl', seems to qualify as an attempt to redefine the relationship between the two on a more personal level. The final excerpt to be presented in this chapter provides another example that shows how the participants use non-task talk to temporarily break out of the narrowly defined institutional frame, and how they manage to get back in.

Excerpt 6.15 is the beginning of an interaction between the station nurse and a resident from the Kansai area (western Japan), who is well-known in Edogawa Care for her characteristic regional accent. The opening is rather unusual, starting with some sort of verbal play on the greeting formula *ohayoo gozaimasu* (Good morning), which by the time the excerpt starts has been exchanged several times with a different accentuation. The first non-task topic

Excerpt 6.15 (#37'9–44)

9	CW	*oHAyoo gozaima*[*su*
		Good morning
10	Res	[*ara ma*
		Oh dear
11		*kuchi ippai kao ippai* [*ya na* ((laughs))=
		mouth covered, face covered
12	CW	[((laughs))
13		=*kazeppoi kara ne,*
		I feel I'm getting a cold, you know
14		*minna ni utsushicha ikenai kara sa*
		and it's no good if I pass it on to everyone
15		(0.7)
16	Res	*kusuri nonderu no?*
		Are you taking medicine?
17	CW	*soo, nonderu no*
		Yes, I do.
18	Res	*nonderu no ee kedo,*
		Medicine is okay,
19		*anta ue nanka kin NA:*[*sai*
		but also put on some more clothes!
20	CW	[*atsukutte:*
		It's hot!
21	Res	*honma nan*
		Really?
22	CW	*ugoiteru to ne*
		When you're moving around
23		(0.5)
24	Res	*na: ase kaku no mo*=
		Right, and sweating is also
25		=*warui ya* [*ne*
		bad, isn't it
26	CW	[*un soo na no* [*yo ne, de soto ni*=
		Uh-huh, that's true, and when I
27	Res	[*un, sore wa*
		Uh-huh, that's
28	CW	=*gomi sute iku to samukut*[*te ne*
		go to throw out the garbage, it's cold
29	Res	[*samukute ne*=
		Cold, isn't it
30	CW	=*demo soo iu toki ue dake*=
		but then I put on
31		=*haotteru kara,* [*chanto*
		my jacket, properly
32	Res	[*sokka*=
		I see
33	CW	=*u:n*=
		Uh-huh

(Continued)

Excerpt 6.15 (Continued)

34	Res	=*daijoobu?*= Okay?
35	CW	=*daijoobu ari*[*gatoo* Okay, thank you
36	Res	[*unn* Uh-huh
37		(1.9, sound of wheelchair footrests unfolded)
38		*kaze hiitara naoran ne,* Once you catch a cold you won't get rid of it
39		*kono goro no ###*[*#n:nakana*[*ka ne:* these days, just like that, you know
40	CW	[*ne::* [*doo shimashoo,* Right, what shall we do?
41		*okimasu ka?* Are you getting up?
42	Res	*u:n, soo, nanji?* Uh-huh, right, what time?
43	CW	*rokuji mawatta kedo* Past six
44	Res	*a, hona okiyoo* Oh, let's get up then

is initiated by the resident in direct succession to the greeting, and partially in overlap with the care worker's last *ohayoo gozaimasu* (lines 9–10). She laughingly comments on the surgical mask the care worker is wearing that day (a quite common phenomenon in Japan also outside healthcare contexts, e.g., Horii 2014), and how it covers most of her face (line 11).

The care worker explains that this is because she feels she is getting a cold, and does not want to 'pass it on to everyone' (lines 13–14). In reaction to this, the resident asks if she is taking medicine, to which the care worker replies in the affirmative (lines 16–17). Interesting about these first couple of lines is how the resident takes advantage of the 'first position' (ten Have 1991: 146) in this non-task talk sequence and how this puts her in charge of determining the further course of the interaction, in a way similar to the nurse call opening discussed in section 5.1 (see excerpt 5.8).

The next utterance by the resident is particularly interesting. While acknowledging that medicine is important, she explicitly takes issue with the care worker's being dressed too lightly, advising her to 'put on some more clothes!' (line 19). She does so using an imperative format and the very informal second person pronoun *anta* (see section 4.1.3). Even if we acknowledge some likely impact of the Kansai dialect, which is known to be more direct than the Japanese spoken in and around Tokyo, this way of telling off the care worker clearly evokes some sort of family relationship that is fundamentally at odds with the participants' institutional roles.

As to the care worker, she eagerly takes up her part in this role play by designing her reply in an almost child-like complaint style: It's hot when you keep moving around (lines 20 and 22), but then you also have to go out into the cold to throw away the garbage (lines 26 and 28) – although, as she dutifully reports, she 'properly' (*chanto*) puts on a jacket on these occasions (lines 30–31). The grievances she shares with the resident here, and the insights she grants her into the institutional 'off limits', imply no minor degree of mutual trust that would appear somewhat out of place if the relationship was defined merely on the basis of the participants' roles as providing and receiving ends in an institutional service encounter.

The sequence continues for a few more lines, in which the resident asks the care worker if she is alright, the care worker confirms and thanks, and the resident reconfirms with a sequence closing third (lines 34–36). At this point, the care worker has started some definite getting-up preparations, as can be understood from the sound of the wheelchair that becomes audible in the pause that follows (line 37). The resident, however, decides to remain in non-task talk mode just a little longer, adding that once you have caught a cold, you will not get rid of it that easily (lines 38–39).

This is the point where the care worker, somewhat forcefully, steps on the brake to get the task work on track. She does so with an emphatically pronounced response token, *ne::* 'Right', delivered in overlap with the resident's yet unfinished turn (lines 39 and 40). Closely in line with Tanaka's (2000: 1171) observations on the multiple functions of *ne*, the way it is used here as a full turn makes it 'a vehicle for reconfirming an agreed point, in the final stages of a discussion on a topic, while simultaneously proposing the termination of further talk on the topic'.

The switch back to task talk follows directly afterwards, and still partially in overlap with the resident's ongoing non-task talk: 'What shall we do? Are you getting up?' (lines 40 and 41). Note that this switch coincides with a stylistic upgrade from non-formal to formal (*shimashoo, okimasu*, see section 4.2), which marks off this new utterance as incongruent with the previous speech. The resident signalises her understanding with *un* and *soo* in the next turn (line 42), and after a brief inquiry about the time agrees to the suggested course of actions. The interaction is in task mode now, and the participants back at their institutionally predefined roles.

Two moments in this excerpt deserve special attention. One is the resident's lengthening of the imperative form *kin NA::sai* in the control act in line 19, where she admonishes the care worker to 'put on some more clothes'. Her 'stretched' pronunciation here seems to express some degree of hesitation about whether the form is appropriate for talking to the care worker. A second noteworthy passage is the 1.9-second pause after the provisional termination of the sequence in line 37. At this point in the interaction, there are two possible directions that could be taken: remain in non-task talk mode or switch into task talk. The pause of almost two seconds seems to suggest that each of the two participants is somewhat unsure about how to continue from here (although the care worker has already started preparing the wheelchair). Both the hesitant imperative form and the intermediate pause suggest a certain degree of insecurity of the interlocutors as to the role they are currently playing, or supposed to play.

6.4　Discussion

This chapter has focused on the most substantial part of the morning care interactions and, in some sense, their very raison d'être: the task work and how it is verbally coordinated by the participants. As Sachweh (2000: 122) has emphasised, the 'main purpose of communication in eldercare is tackling the tasks', and this definitely holds for the present data, too. Accordingly, the interactions abound with elements that I have referred to by the summarising label 'task talk': requests and other control acts, inquiries about things to be done, the task transition marker *hai,*, and various types of heave-hoes. The analysis has shown how these verbal activities are closely linked to a 'baseline of physical activities' (Engbersen 2013: 1–2) that keeps running in the background, and thus fulfil an important coordinative function. Since the participants are working through the tasks together, they must make sure that their actions are optimally attuned to each other. This is the basic purpose of task talk, and arguably the sole reason for its occurrence.

One general observation about the task talk elements discussed is that they show the care workers' strong grip on the performance of the activities. It is them, rather than the residents, who make most of the requests; it is them who call for confirmation, more than once where deemed necessary, and who have the last word by 'confirming confirmation' with a sequence closing third; it is them who acknowledge the completion of a running task and the beginning of a new one with *hai,*; and it is them who do most of the 'heave-hoeing' that comes with the task activities.

While task talk clearly dominates the morning care in Edogawa Care, we have also seen that the participants frequently find other things to tell each other as they work their way from bed to breakfast. The 107 interactions contain a total of 163 non-task talk sequences, in which a greater variety of topics are discussed. Most of them are closely linked to the here and now of institutional everyday life, such as the previous night, today's events, or other residents. With regard to the initiation of non-task talk, there appears to be a general preference by the care workers to talk about things other than those pertaining to their in-group. We have seen that such topics are brought up almost exclusively by the residents, and as excerpt 6.11 has shown, may remain unattended to by a care worker.

On the other hand, the excerpts discussed in the later part of the chapter reveal that both resident and care worker occasionally talk about themselves and their non-institutional background at some length, thereby disclosing no minor amount of personal information. This echoes Heritage and Clayman's (2010: 35) observation that '"ordinary conversation" can emerge in almost any seemingly institutional context'. And while Grainger (2004b: 486) holds that even such instances of 'personal discourse' are essentially aimed at getting the tasks done, the example presented in excerpt 6.14 suggests that this is not necessarily so. When talking about his experiences at vocational college, the care worker's eagerness to get his story told clearly gets in the way of a smooth task performance. He is working while talking, rather than talking while working, and it is the resident who has to direct his attention back to the tasks, two times in succession. The care worker in this scene presents himself as considerably 'non-professional' (Nussbaum 1991: 157), though not necessarily in a bad sense (see also Coupland 2000: 20).

In fact, many previous studies have emphasised the favourable effects of non-task talk elements in care communication. As Suwa (1996: 20) points out in a Japanese care communication primer, chit-chat (*zatsudan*) is an act of care in and of itself. Gibb (1990: 14) in her research in Australia has observed that the occurrence of non-task talk facilitates 'a fluid transition between roles which reflect unequal status – such as giver and receiver of instruction, explanation, support and so on – to one of mutual involvement of participants of equal standing'. Likewise, Matsumoto (2011: 163) holds that 'rather than keeping the rigid division of caregiver and care recipient – or person in full health vs. person in declining health – adopting various roles suitable for different situations can encourage more satisfying communication'. There is some chance that the stories the participants are telling each other in the examples discussed – about accidents with sewing machines, astonishing discoveries at college, and upcoming colds – may have similar positive effects, for both participants involved.

One structural problem of non-task talk sequences is that they are vulnerable to being cancelled by task talk at virtually any interactional moment. This requires some considerable coordinative extra work by the participants involved. Both care worker and care recipient seem to share an overall understanding that task talk overrules non-task talk, and they frequently show an awareness of the problem by designing their verbal returns to a task in a minimally intrusive way. As excerpts 6.13 and 6.14 suggest, a soliloquy-like preparation, often delivered in sotto voce, appears to be a feasible device to do so. As a result of such efforts, task talk and non-task talk may run simultaneously for quite a number of turns. On the other hand, there are also a couple of ways to explicitly mark off an urgent task talk sequence from the running non-task talk. These include use of the task transition marker *hai,* and shifts from plain to formal style. The occurrence of this great variety of – and in part quite contrary – devices testifies to the delicacy of balancing the urgency of a current task with the continuing relevance of a running non-task talk sequence.

Another problem is how to reactivate suspended non-task talk once the necessary bits of task talk have been delivered. The analysis has shown that the participants can handle this in more and less 'fluent' ways. In excerpt 6.12, the resident and care worker's understanding about the proper point of re-entry into the pending non-task talk so precisely agrees that both start to speak at virtually the same moment – the resident with the sequel to her story and the care worker with a backchannel token that signalises his re-availability as story recipient. By contrast, in excerpt 6.13, which occurs only a number of seconds later, the participants' construal of their interactional 'you are here' has become slightly disconnected, and it takes a number of turns to re-establish a stable speaker–hearer relationship.

The organisation of multiactivity in social interaction is a problem we are only beginning to understand (Haddington et al. 2014a, Oshima and Streeck 2015). The analysis in this chapter has shown how the physical activities generate a number of verbalisations, here called task talk, that serve to assure a coordinated performance of the care tasks. This 'matrix exchange' (Kuiper and Flindall 2000: 192) is comparatively easy to handle because the talking and the physical activities go 'hand in hand' and will not get in the way of each other. However, if the verbal channel becomes occupied by what we have referred to as non-task talk, the participants must switch 'from simultaneous to consecutive ordering' (Keisanen et al. 2014: 109) to coordinate the two separate, functionally disjunct lines of talk. Despite the non-availability of visual information, the present chapter has tried to capture how residents and care workers manage to handle this in their talk at work.

It is a matter of fact that such coordination problems between task talk and non-task talk will show up only in cases where non-task talk occurs in the first place. When there is nothing else the participants have to say, the only thing the task talk will compete with is silence. While this may be the smoothest way to coordinate the tasks, it is most likely not the best possible way of giving, and receiving, care.

7 Tempo

One of my earliest impressions when listening through the recordings was that many of the interactions were characterised by some sort of hurriedness in the speech of the care workers, which frequently seemed to clash with the residents' considerably slower pace. It proved somewhat difficult, though, to determine how exactly this impression came about, and where it could be pinpointed in the data. It was only after I had finished transcribing and started various other parts of the analysis that I was able to identify some recurrent patterns indicative of the differences between the 'operation speed' of the care workers and the tempo that the residents seemed to prefer.

Peripherally, we have already come across this problem on several occasions throughout the previous chapters: when discussing a style downgrade from a beautified to a non-beautified form in chapter 4 (excerpt 4.7), noticing instances of 'talking while leaving' in chapter 5 (excerpt 5.15), and analysing the repetition of first pair parts in inquiries and other sequences, as discussed in chapter 6 (excerpt 6.5). The aim of this chapter is to have a more focused look on how the tempo differences between residents and staff manifest themselves in the small print of the interactional give and take. The following three phenomena will be discussed: overlaps (section 7.1), multiple sayings (section 7.2), and subsequent versions (section 7.3).

7.1 Overlaps

One basic rule of thumb about talk in interaction is that only one person speaks at a time (Sacks et al. 1974). This being said, instances of two or more people producing simultaneous speech can and do occur. In their seminal paper on turn-taking, Sacks et al. (1974) identify various conditions that commonly involve temporary overlaps of two concurrent turns. These include instances where a 'next speaker' misprojects the length of a running turn and starts while the 'previous speaker' has not finished yet, or where more than one speaker self-selects as next speaker after a completed turn, as a result of which two or more turns get launched at the same time. In addition, there are what Schegloff (2000: 6) calls 'licensed or mandated productions of simultaneous talk' such as laughter, greetings, and leave-takings, where overlaps are fully intended and in fact the most unmarked form of turn-taking. While such cases do not challenge another speaker's right to complete her or his turn – and are not normally treated that way by the participants – previous studies have frequently identified other instances of overlaps that seem to do just that (e.g., West and Zimmerman 1977).

In an attempt to capture the problem in a more precise way, Schegloff (1987, 2002) has distinguished between overlaps and interruptions. The former refer 'generically to any case of more than one party speaking at a time', whereas the latter term is 'reserved (roughly) for starts by a second speaker while another is speaking and is not near possible completion' (Schegloff 1987: 85). How interruptive an overlap is – and how to make a distinction between the two – has remained a controversial issue (e.g., Jefferson 1984a, Goldberg 1990, Murata 1994, Bilmes 1997), but one that will concern us here only peripherally. What the analysis in this section aims to show is how such overlaps may indicate differing tempo preferences by the speakers producing them.

Overlaps have been a frequent topic in research on doctor–patient interactions. An early example is West's (1984) study from a family practice centre in the southern US. West observed that male doctors in this setting would interrupt their patients much more frequently than vice versa (though for female doctors, the situation was largely reversed). Similar observations about an unequal share of interruptions between doctors and patients were made in various other studies (e.g., Beckman and Frankel 1984, Marvel et al. 1999), while research challenging these findings also exists (e.g., Street and Buller 1988, Irish and Hall 1995).

Despite a large number of studies on overlaps, it seems that the relationship between interruptions and interactional tempo so far has gone largely unexplored. An exception is Li and his colleagues' (2008) research on interactions between medical practitioners and patients in a Canadian hospital. Correlating the number and types of interruptions with patient satisfaction, as evaluated in a subsequent questionnaire survey, they found that there was a statistically significant relationship between the number of a patient's 'unsuccessful interruptions' that did not stop a doctor from aborting his running turn, and that patient's assessment that 'my doctor seemed in a hurry' (Li et al. 2008: 420). That 'being in a hurry' does not necessarily translate into getting things done more quickly is one of the main findings in Menz and Al-Roubaie's (2008) study on doctor–patient communication in an Austrian healthcare setting. They show that the more often a doctor non-supportively interrupts a patient, the longer an interaction will take.

In her study on resident–staff communication in a German care facility, Sachweh identifies a specific type of overlap that she classifies as a threat to a resident's face. An example from her data is an interaction where a resident observes that they are *fast fertich* 'almost done' with the morning care, and begins saying *das übrige, äh* 'the rest, uh', at which point the care worker continues in her stead, saying *das erledigen wir jetzt* 'that we'll do now' (Sachweh 2003: 157, transcription slightly simplified). Though Sachweh states that cases like this are rather rare, and largely confined to interactions with speech-impaired residents, she emphasises that such 'premature intervention', even if well-intended, can 'communicate a feeling of incompetence to the residents' (Sachweh 2000: 181). With respect to tempo, she speculates that this type of overlap arises from a care worker's impatience when a resident's running turn is not completed 'quickly enough' (Sachweh 2003: 157).

7.1.1 Non-problematic vs. problematic overlaps

We have encountered various instances of overlaps in the previous chapters: during terminal exchanges in closings (section 5.2.3), in second pair parts of heave-hoes (section 6.1.4), and when a switch from non-task talk to task talk is necessary (section 6.3.). A simple count of pairs of square brackets in the corpus shows that the 107 interactions contain more than 1,250 such instances, indicating an average of almost 12 overlaps per interaction. As a matter of fact, most of these are just the common 'driftwood' of spoken interaction, and do not point to any tempo problems whatsoever. Excerpt 7.1, which presents a brief passage from a non-task talk sequence about bathing, is an example to bring this point home.

As mentioned in section 6.2, bathing is one of the most favourable non-task topics residents and staff talk about during the morning care routines. The resident in this excerpt has just told the care worker that last Monday, she had to wait for her turn until after noon. The care worker in line 38 explains this with the fact that on Mondays, the male residents bathe first, knowledge of which is signalised by the resident's partially overlapping confirmation in line 39. After a pause of 1.9 seconds, both participants start to speak simultaneously (and incidentally with the same word, lines 41 and 42), but the resident quickly aborts her turn and lets the care worker finish first. After that, she has a second go with what she was about to say (line 43), but again is unable to finish, due to another overlap with the care worker's speech (line 44).

The excerpt contains a total of three overlaps. The first one (lines 38 and 39) results from an 'acknowledgement token' (Jefferson 1984b) by the resident

Excerpt 7.1 (#84'38–44)

38	CW	*getsuyoobi wa otoko no hito kara da*[*kara ne*
		Because on Mondays it's the men first
39	Res	[*un un*
		Uh, uh
40		(1.9)
41		[*kyoo:*
		Today
42	CW	[*kyoo wa daijoobu yo*
		Today it's alright
43	Res	*kyoo: wa onna* [*ga sa/*
		Today it's women fir/
44	CW	[*onna ga saki dakara ne*
		because women are first, right

towards the end of the care worker's running statement that 'on Mondays it's the men first'. The second overlap (lines 41 and 42) occurs after the 1.9-second pause that has temporarily set the turn-taking machinery on hold. Unsure about who is going to speak next, the two participants simultaneously self-select to start a new turn. Both the first and the second overlap are entirely unproblematic and, if anything, show how well the operational speeds of the two participants are attuned to one another.

The third overlap, in lines 43 and 44, deserves some more attention. Here, it seems that the resident's attempt to display her institutional knowledge that 'Today it's women first' is 'taken over' and finished by the care worker in her stead. There is clearly no misprojection of turn length because the resident's turn is nowhere near completion by the time the overlap starts. It is a very similar case to the one observed in Sachweh's (2003: 157) study, as described above. Though we may consider this a well-intended attempt at 'collaborative completion' (Liddicoat 2004), or what Murata (1994) calls 'co-operative interruption', we could also – or perhaps simultaneously – follow Sachweh's interpretation in arguing that the care worker's 'pre-emptive completion' (Lerner 2004) of what the resident was just about to say is an attempt to accelerate things by verbally helping the resident along. In this case, it would in fact be indicative of a difference in interactional speed.

7.1.2 'Overdue' second pair parts

Whereas the example just discussed remains somewhat ambivalent, there are other instances of overlaps in the data that clearly hint at substantial tempo differences between resident and care worker. These seem to be particularly frequent in the opening phase of an interaction, perhaps owing to the fact that, as described in section 5.1, many of the residents are not yet fully 'in play' (Schegloff 1968: 1086) by the time the interaction starts. The example presented in excerpt 7.2 is prototypical in this respect. The care worker enters the room, opens the resident's bed curtains (line 1) and addresses her with a combined summons and greeting (line 2). After a pause of 0.8 seconds, the resident delivers her reply to the greeting (line 4).

The overlap occurs just here, between the resident's completion of the greeting with a second pair part and the care worker's launch of a new first pair part.

Excerpt 7.2 (#57'1–5)

1	CW	((enters room, opens bed curtains))
2		*LN-san ohayoo*
		LN-san, good morning
3		(0.8)
4	Res	*o[hayoo*
		Good morning.
5	CW	[*nanji ni okiteru?*
		What time are you getting up?

Crucial for the understanding of the overlap is the preceding pause in line 3, which opens up where the care worker is waiting for the resident's reply to his greeting. However, by the time that reply finally comes, the care worker has already prepared a new turn, which now starts almost simultaneously with the resident's. While on the surface this looks like just another case of simultaneous self-selection after a pause, it is clearly different from the example presented in excerpt 7.1 (lines 41 and 42) in that the sequence has not been formally closed yet, and the resident's possible reply at this point is still pending.

The exchange in excerpt 7.2 suggests that the care worker expects the second pair part to his greeting to be delivered within a certain time frame, or what Jefferson (1989: 170) calls 'tolerance interval'. If that fails to happen, he considers it fit to proceed to the next stage without having his greeting reciprocated. This concurs with Kitamoto's (2006: 55) observations that adjacency pairs in her Japanese care data frequently failed to evolve because the care worker decided to move on when there was no immediate reaction by a resident. With respect to the present data, it may also be one major reason for the fact that a care worker's greeting frequently remains unreciprocated by a resident, as we have seen in chapter 5 (see section 5.1.1).

As to the resident, her eventual delivery of the second pair part shows that she is well aware of the sequential relevance of her reply at this point. However, the fact that she replies outside the time frame deemed appropriate by the care worker suggests that she has a different idea regarding the operational tempo of the greeting exchange as a whole. The resulting 'collision' of the two turns – a second pair part that refers back to a still relevant first pair part, and a new first pair part that cancels that very relevance – can be read as a manifestation of these disparate time expectancies.

Another example, again from the opening phase, is presented in excerpt 7.3. It is a brief sequence about the reason for the encounter that starts with the care worker asking the resident the standard question about getting up (line 8). This time, the resident's reply (line 9) is delivered without any delay in second pair part position – which would formally suffice to complete the sequence. However, as in other cases previously described (e.g., excerpts 5.2 and 6.4), the resident's reply is reconfirmed by the care worker with a sequence closing third (line 10).

Excerpt 7.3 (#22'8–11)

8	CW	*okiru?* Get up?
9	Res	*o[kiru* Get up
10	CW	*[ne, hai* Right, okay
11	Res	*hai* Okay

Noteworthy about this third turn is that it is delivered largely in overlap with the resident's reply. In other words, the care worker acknowledges the resident's second pair part already in advance of its actual production. This reveals a somewhat problematic presumption that an affirmative reply was the only possible choice at this stage, and that a rejection was not even considered an option.

In addition, and most relevant for the topic of this chapter, the timing of the care worker's sequence closing third adds hurriedness to the interaction through the delivery of a new turn at a time when the previous one has hardly begun. As in the previous example, the care worker here seems to be moving along with a considerably higher speed than the resident, to an extent that she is almost 'lapping' her interactional co-runner at this point. In effect, however, the collision of the two turns necessitates an additional acknowledgement by the resident, in line 11, just to be sure. Put differently, the care worker's efforts to speed up things actually extend a sequence of minimally two turns into one of four. We will come back to this contradictory effect in the course of this chapter.

In closing this section, it needs to be reemphasised that overlaps are an entirely common feature of naturally occurring interaction, and indeed part of what makes it natural in the first place. The examples presented in excerpt 7.1 have been chosen to show just that. In this respect, the mere number of overlaps in an interaction has little – if anything – to say about the quality of the communication as a whole. On the other hand, the examples subsequently discussed suggest that when an overlap results from the simultaneous delivery of a resident's 'overdue' second pair part and a care worker's new first pair part (excerpt 7.2) or sequence closing third (excerpt 7.3), this can be taken as a reliable indication of the participants' differing tempo preferences.

7.2 Multiple sayings

A second point of interest with respect to the interactional tempo is repetitions in the speech of the care workers, many of which occur within a single turn. Such within-turn reiterations have been examined more closely by Stivers (2004), who refers to them as 'multiple sayings' and characterises them as follows: They '(a) involve a full unit of talk being said multiple times, (b) are said by the same speaker, (c) have a similar segmental character, (d) happen immediately in succession, and (e) are done under a single intonation contour' (Stivers 2004: 261). Multiple sayings can consist of single lexical items such as 'no no no no:', but can also repeat phrasal or sentential items, as in 'Right there=right there=right there' or 'Waidaminit waidaminit' (Stivers 2004: 265–267, transcription slightly simplified). One main function of multiple sayings as observed by Stivers (2004: 280) is to 'convey that the speaker has found the prior speaker's course of action to have perseverated needlessly and proposes that the course of action be halted' (Stivers 2004: 280). Similar phenomena of reduplication, both with similar and with rather distinct functions, have been examined in other languages (Wierzbicka 1991: chapter 7, Israeli 1997, Golato and Fagyal 2008, Heinemann 2009b, Keevallik 2010).

Multiple sayings, though not by this name, have been identified as one common feature in aviation communication. Sassen (2005) in a study on 'crisis talk' between pilots and the tower frequently finds such items in situations of danger and high psychological stress. She categorises them according to utterance type into directives ('the lower one, the lower one, the lower one, the lower one'), assertives ('open open') and expressives ('Oh my god, oh my god'), but observes that especially repetitions of directives 'might be interpreted as a functional shift by which the directive obtains some qualities of an expressive' (Sassen 2005: 156–157). Though this observation is not developed in more detail, Sassen's main point here seems to be that multiple sayings of a directive in such highly precarious situations are not primarily used to provide tailor-made instructions for a requested action, but also serve to 'let off steam' in the face of a critical situation that the speaker is not able to directly influence.

In the context of eldercare, the occurrence of multiple sayings is briefly discussed by Furuta and Horie (2011: 248), who identify utterances such as *koko koko* 'here, here' or *suwatte suwatte* 'sit down, sit down' as instances of elderspeak. Posenau (2014: 100) in his study in a German dementia care facility observes that within-turn repetitions are used by the care workers to 'brake' unwanted or premature activities by a resident. One example he presents features a resident who has just been brought back from the toilet to her room and is about to sit down there. However, the care worker has not yet properly positioned the chair and, in order to prevent a fall, now tries to stop the resident's action by producing a multiple saying of the phrase *ein moment* 'one moment'. This way of using multiple sayings corresponds with Stivers' (2004) observations that they function to put another speaker's action to a halt. The difference is that, in the case presented by Posenau, the action is not a verbal but a physical one.

7.2.1 *Repeated material*

Multiple sayings in my data share all five criteria outlined by Stivers (2004), and have two more characteristics: They are exclusively produced by the care workers, and occur only in task talk. As in Sassen's (2005) study, they frequently serve to provide 'quick' directions about a required next action, but are also used as attempts to make a resident stop what he or she is doing or about to do, in a similar way as observed by Posenau (2014). In both cases, they qualify as control acts (see section 6.1.1).

One type of lexical material that is frequently repeated within turns is 'items' belonging to the resident. These include parts of a resident's body (e.g., *te* 'hand', *ashi* 'feet') and things to be 'attached' to it (e.g., *kutsushita* 'socks', *ireba* 'dentals'). Another favourable material for repetitions is deictic expressions (e.g., *kotchi* 'here', *gyaku* 'other way round', etc.). They specify the direction of a requested movement, and thus constitute an implicit request to perform that movement. As we will see, reiterative mentioning of these types of items within one turn, usually in quick succession, conveys some sort of urgency that appears to be intended to speed up a resident's 'delivery' of the requested action.

Table 7.1 Repeated material in multiple sayings

Type	Gloss	Transcript location
(1) Resident's 'items'		
te te te	hand (3x)	(#1'31)
ashi ashi	foot/feet (2x)	(#85'157) (see excerpt 7.4)
ireba ireba	dentals (2x)	(#15'93f)
kutsushita kutsushita	socks (2x)	(#64'86)
(2) Deictic expressions		
kotchi kotchi kotchi kotchi	here (4x)	(#1'29)
sotchi sotchi sotchi	there (3x)	(#74'137)
gyaku gyaku	other way round (2x)	(#74'38)
ue ue ue	up (3x)	(#74'94)
(3) Brakes		
chie chechejeje	no (5x)	(#47'74) (see excerpt 7.5)
chottomat chodo matchodo matte	wait a second (3x)	(#64'79)
abunai abunai abunan	caution (3x)	(#85'290)
chotto madayo madayo	not yet (2x)	(#85'168) (see excerpt 7.4)

A third common constituent of multiple sayings is expressions used to communicate a warning. This, too, can be done by repetition of single words (e.g., *abunai* 'caution'), but may also involve syntactically more complex material. Irrespective of length and complexity, all multiple sayings in this 'brake' category are intended to prevent or halt a resident's action. Table 7.1 lists examples of the three types of multiple sayings from the data. The next section takes a closer look at how they function in interactions.

7.2.2   *Multiple sayings in interaction*

Excerpt 7.4 contains two examples of multiple sayings in use. The participants have just moved to the toilet, where the care worker has made the resident stand up from her wheelchair and asked her to hold tight to the handrail. The next thing that needs to be done is positioning the resident's feet in a way that will make it possible for her to move over and sit on the toilet. This is where the first multiple saying occurs, a repetition of the word *ashi* 'feet' (line 157). Note that, following Stivers (2004), the multiple saying does not include the first *ashi* because it is not done within the same intonation contour but delivered separately. In other words, we have the common control act format of a (single word) noun phrase instruction (see section 6.1.1), followed by a multiple saying with the same lexical item. In agreement with the usual pattern, the requested action itself is performed by the resident without verbalisation, and then acknowledged by the care worker with *un* (line 158).

Excerpt 7.4 (#85'156–170)

156	CW	LN-*san ashi*, LN-*san*, feet
157		*ashi ashi*, feet feet,
158		*un, yoisho* Uh-huh ((heave-ho))
159		(1.4)
160		*ii kana?* Alright?
161		(0.8)
162		*isu hikimasu yo* I pull away the (wheel)chair now
163	Res	*a:* Uh
164		(2.2)
165	CW	*un oroshimasu=* Uh-huh, I pull down your pants
166		*=uo:::* Uh-oh!
167		(1.0)
168		*chotto madayo madayo* Wait, not yet not yet
169		(2.1)
170		*hai, do::h zo* Okay, here you go

Though difficult to confirm without video data, this acknowledgment suggests that the care worker's repeats continue just to the point where the resident starts reacting as requested. This mechanism would also explain the differing number of repeats we find in the data. As can be seen in Table 7.1, there is a range from between two to five items in a turn, which might reflect differences in 'reaction time' by the residents. This would be an alternative explanation to Stivers (2004: 291), who suggests that the frequency of a repeated item in her – admittedly different – data set may be related to 'the strength or intensity of the action'.

Back in our excerpt, the next thing that needs to be done is move away the empty wheelchair and pull down the resident's trousers, as announced by the care worker in lines 162 and 165, respectively. We do not know what exactly happens after that, but the care worker's latched *uo:::* exclamation in line 166 suggests it was something unexpected. Briefly after that, she produces a second multiple saying, *madayo madayo* 'not yet not yet' (line 168), obviously in reaction to the resident's premature attempt to sit down. It takes a few more moments to complete all necessary preparations, after which the action can finally be performed. It is verbally coordinated by the care worker with *hai,* and an extraordinarily lengthened *do::h zo* 'here you go', articulation of which seems to be closely mapped onto the action of sitting the resident down on the toilet seat.

The two multiple sayings in this excerpt do different but related things. The first one is an attempt to accelerate a requested action ('move feet') by repeatedly calling for its performance. The second one does just the opposite: keeping the resident from performing an action ('sit down') because it is considered premature at this point and a possible threat to the resident's safety, just like in the example presented by Posenau (2014: 100).

That multiple sayings of the 'brake' type do not necessarily relate to safety issues can be understood from the example presented in excerpt 7.5, a different interaction at the toilet from a slightly later stage of the routines. The resident has already moved over to sit on the toilet, with the care worker now dressing her. In the excerpt, the first task the care worker announces is inserting the resident's feet into some piece of clothing, performed during the 35 seconds of silence that follow (lines 66 and 67). It is not entirely clear what the care worker's next utterance refers to (line 68), but somewhere towards the end of the ensuing silence, the resident seems to make an effort to stand up. That is where he tells her that she should not do so yet (line 70) because he wants to finish the dressing first (line 72). The two multiple sayings occur briefly after that, in line 74, which is quite packed with repetitions: two times *te* 'hand', followed by a very quickly pronounced chain of the verb *chigau* (literally, 'be different/wrong'). It is delivered a total of five times in a row, thereby increasingly dissolving into a mere string of affricates.

Excerpt 7.5 (#47'66–77)

66	CW	*ashi ireyo*
		Let's put in your feet
67		(35.5)
68		*un ii yo hazusu kara*
		Uh-huh, never mind I'll pull it out anyway
69		(9.5)
70		*chotto mada tatanai de,*
		Don't stand up yet
71		(0.3)
72		*yoofu/uwagi kigae(ru)kara*
		Because we'll put on your clo/jacket
73		(0.4)
74		*te te chie chechejeje*
		Hand hand no nononnonno
75		(2.0)
76		*un, kotchi mo*
		Right, this one too
77		(5.0)

As in the previous excerpt, the care worker's multiple sayings calls for a quick reaction by the resident to do one thing ('produce hand') and not do another (most likely, 'produce wrong hand'). And here, too, both multiple sayings function to get the resident's movements in tune with the tempo of the care worker. The difference is that, in the present case, the action the care worker tries to 'brake' does not seem to involve any safety issues, as there is no real danger in producing one hand instead of the other in this situation. This shows that while multiple sayings may be an unavoidable and totally justified device to protect a resident from falling or prevent other accidents, even the 'brake' type in many cases seems to result first and foremost from a care worker's perceived need to hurry, dictating when, in what order, and at what speed the tasks are to be performed. Many multiple sayings in the data thus seem to be motivated more by impatience than by real urgency.

7.3 Subsequent versions

Repetitions of previously used material are not confined to one-word instructions within single turns, but can take the shape of whole turns. This phenomenon has already been recognised by Schegloff (1968) in his seminal paper on conversational openings. When discussing the summons part at the beginning of an interaction, he observes that '[i]f one party issues an S[ummons] and no A[nswer] occurs, that provides the occasion for repetition of the S'. This means that 'the non-occurrence of the A is seen by the summoner as its official absence and its official absence provides him with adequate grounds for repetition of the S' (Schegloff 1968: 1084).

Schegloff further holds that these types of repetitions do not necessarily constitute identical versions of each other, but 'may change over some string of repetitions'. Examples he quotes include shifts from 'Mommy . . . Mommy' to 'Mum . . . Mum' or from a ring of the doorbell to a knock on the door (Schegloff 1968: 1085).

Such 'successive utterances', as Schegloff (1968: 1085) calls them, do not only occur in summons–answer sequences, but can be found in many other sequence types. Davidson (1984) examines a greater variety of invitations and offers by a first speaker that do not entail an immediate response by a second speaker. Such silences after a first pair part are well-known in conversation analysis as foreshadowing some sort of non-acceptance by the second speaker (Pomerantz 1984a). In order to deal with the problem, the first speaker in the data examined by Davidson (1984: 107) offers what she calls a 'subsequent version' of the initial FPP, which serves to 'provide a next place for a response', and hopefully a positive one. Though only some of the subsequent versions examined by Davidson involve material recycled from the initial version, the mechanism she identifies closely resembles the turn structure of the examples to be discussed here. That is why her term is used in this study.

A slightly different type of subsequent version has been discussed in Sassen's (2005) previously mentioned study of air traffic communication. With reference to Gibbon's (1981) analysis of international amateur radio talk, she identifies so-called 'uptake loops' in her data. These result from a first speaker's question ('Did you ever take it out of here?') or other utterance in first pair part position, replied to by a second speaker with some sort of request for clarification ('Huh?'). In reaction, the first speaker delivers a subsequent version ('Have you ever taken it out of here?'), to which the second speaker – if properly understood this time – will then provide an appropriate reply ('Hadn't till now') as the (delayed) second pair part (Sassen 2005: 161).

In the care context, a comparable use of subsequent versions has been observed by Posenau (2014: 79–80) in his study in a German eldercare facility. He found that care workers in his data frequently repeated their opening greeting. In one example he presents, the standard greeting *guten morgen* 'Good morning' is first delivered by a care worker on entering the room. For lack of a resident's uptake, it is repeated by the care worker two times, the second time shortened into *morgen* 'Morning'. An even longer stretch of repeats is discussed by Akiya (2008: 62–64) in a study on resident–staff interaction in a Japanese day care centre. Structurally speaking, both examples bear some resemblance with Sassen's uptake loops, except for the non-trivial fact that, as in Davidson's data, the subsequent versions are entirely unsolicited here.

7.3.1   Non-uptake loops

In the present study, we have come across similar turn repeats, for instance, when examining inquiry sequences in section 6.1.2 (see excerpt 6.5) or when discussing the properties of the opening phase in section 5.1. In this latter case, we have looked at excerpt 5.3, which is reproduced here as excerpt 7.6.

Relevant to the present discussion is the care worker's greeting in line 4, her slightly shortened repetition of it in line 6, and the resident's reply in line 7. The utterance in line 4 is a first pair part that makes a reply by the resident a

Excerpt 7.6 (#17'1–7)

1	CW	((enters room, opens bed curtains))
2		LN-*sa:n*
		LN-*san*
3		(1.3)
4		*ohayoo gozaimasu*
		Good morning
5		(1.8)
6		*ohayoo*
		Morning
7	Res	(°*ohayo*°)
		Morning

relevant next action. However, as no such action occurs during the 1.8 seconds that follow, the care worker repeats her greeting in line 6. Note that we find the same shortening of the original material (*ohayoo gozaimasu* > *ohayoo*) as in Posenau's German data (*guten morgen* > *morgen*). The subsequent version by the care worker here marks the resident's second pair part as missing, and calls for a repair of this "apparent non-response" (Antaki et al. 2016: 617). And this is indeed what happens, in line 7, where the resident finally provides the requested reply to the care worker's greeting. This formally completes the sequence and allows the interaction to proceed to the next stage.

In some cases, subsequent versions occur more than once in succession. An example is excerpt 7.7, which is another sequence from an opening phase. Unlike in the previous excerpt, the greeting exchange here proceeds very smoothly, with the resident's second pair part delivered in direct adjacency to (and, in fact, partially in overlap with) the care worker's first pair part of the greeting (lines 2 and 3). The turn-taking machinery gets somewhat stuck when the care worker moves on to the reason for the encounter by asking the resident if she would like to get up (line 5). Receiving no direct reply, she repeats her question twice before the resident reacts with an affirmative response (line 11). In other words, as sketched in excerpt 7.7, the original FPP in line 5 for lack of the resident's direct uptake becomes reissued two times in slightly different formats: as FPP' in line 7, and as FPP" in line 9. As a result of these two 'non-uptake loops', the resident's eventual delivery

Excerpt 7.7 (#84'1–12)

1	CW	((enters room, yawns))	
2		*ohayoo gozaimasu*[:: Good morning	
3	Res	[*ohayoo gozaimasu* Good morning	
4		(1.0)	
5	CW	*okimasu ka?* Are you getting up?	(FPP)
6		(1.5)	
7		*okimasu:?* You're getting up?	(FPP')
8		(1.0)	
9		*okiru?* Get up?	(FPP")
10		(0.4)	
11	Res	*okiru=* Get up.	(SPP)
12	CW	=*un* Uh-huh	(SCT)

of the second pair part in line 11 is now considerably remote from the care worker's original first pair part in line 3.

A closer look at the original FPP and its subsequent versions reveals two noteworthy features. First, similar to the example in excerpt 7.6, the turn is not repeated in exactly the same format, but is slightly downgraded both in style and in morphosyntactic complexity. The first time the care worker asks the resident about getting up (line 5), she does so using the verb in formal style and with question marker *ka* attached. When she reissues her question as FPP', she drops the question marker in favour of a pure intonation question. For FPP'', she further downgrades from the formal to the non-formal style (*okimasu* > *okiru*). We have observed a similar type of stylistic downgrade when discussing the shift from *o-toire* to *toire* in section 4.3 (see excerpt 4.7; for a similar case, see Nishizaka 2007: 56). Schegloff (2004) refers to such omissible material as 'dispensables'. A comparable phenomenon has been observed by Craven and Potter (2010: 433) when analysing multiple directives during family dinner interactions.

The second point is the length of the pauses between and after the repeated turns. The first pause (line 6), between the original FPP and its first subsequent version, takes a total of 1.5 seconds. The second pause (line 8), which opens up between the first and the second subsequent version, is considerably shorter, with only 1.0 seconds.

Taken together, the downgrading of the turns and the decreasing length of the pauses conveys a growing impatience on the part of the care worker. It seems that the combination of shorter turns and shorter slots for possible turn insertion increases the 'response pressure' (Stivers and Rossano 2010: 23) on the resident to come up with the pending second pair part, which she eventually does, in line 11. Also note that the care worker's sequence closing third in line 12 is directly latched to the resident's reply. This way of driving the interaction along by compressing the space between turns closely resembles the overlap phenomena discussed in section 7.1 (see excerpt 7.3), and can be taken as another indication of the care worker's hurriedness.

7.3.2   Missing vs. missed second pair parts

A most striking phenomenon is the occurrence of subsequent versions even in cases where a second pair part has already been delivered. The passage in excerpt 7.8 provides an example. It starts with the care worker's suggestion to turn the resident's bed light on (line 82), followed by three subsequent versions of this first pair part, indicated as FPP' (line 85), FPP'' (line 87), and FPP''' (line 89). As in the previous excerpt, there is both a shortening of the turns (except for FPP''', which is an exact replication of FPP', most likely because no further trimming of the one word item *denki* was possible) and an overall shortening of the pauses between these turns, from 0.8 seconds (line 86), to 0.4 seconds (line 88), to a negative value, as the overlap of lines 89 and 90 shows.

Excerpt 7.8 (#84'82–92)

82	CW	LN-*san denki tsu*[*kemasho*	(FPP)
		LN-*san*, let's switch on the light	
83	Res	[*hai*	(SPP)
		Okay	
84		(0.6)	
85	CW	*denki tsukeyoo ka*	(FPP')
		Shall we switch on the light?	
86		(0.8)	
87		*denki*	(FPP'')
		Light	
88		(0.4)	
89		*denki tsukeyoo* [*ka*	(FPP''')
		Shall we switch on the light?	
90	Res	[*un,* [*un*	(SPP')
		Uh, uh	
91	CW	[*un*	(SCT)
		Uh-huh	
92		((light on))	

What substantially differs from the excerpts discussed so far is that the care worker's original FPP in line 82 is in fact immediately attended to by the resident, with a corresponding SPP in line 83. Though this response is clearly audible on tape, it apparently goes unnoticed by the care worker. One likely reason for this is that the resident delivers her reply in complete overlap with the care worker's running FPP, directly after the latter has produced the main lexical item of her turn, *denki* (light). This suffices for the resident to (correctly) project the intended meaning of the care worker's utterance, and come up with a quick response. Note that in contrast to the examples discussed in section 7.1, the overlap here is produced by the resident rather than by the care worker, perhaps in an attempt to speed up things on her part, too. However that may be, her reply does not register with the care worker as intended. This results in the common series of non-uptake loops, which only comes to an end after the resident provides a second SPP, indicated in the transcript as SPP' (line 90). The care worker acknowledges this with a sequence closing third (line 91), directly after which the light goes on.

As this example shows, the care worker's attempts to speed up things through turn repetition can factually result in time loss. In her hurry, she fails to notice the resident's delivery of the pending SPP at the time when it first occurs. The resident's reaction is not missing – it has been missed. The subsequent attempt to fix something that is in fact not broken entails some substantial interactional extra work, both for the care worker, who keeps producing subsequent versions of her original FPP, and for the resident, who has to deliver her SPP twice in order to move the interaction on to the next stage.

The example presented in excerpt 7.8 may appear quite exceptional. However, a look through the transcripts reveals that there is a total of no less than 11 clearly identifiable cases in which a care worker produces one or more subsequent versions of an FPP when a resident's SPP has already been delivered. This means that we find such interactional detours in about one in ten morning care exchanges, suggesting that they are in fact more common than one might expect.

7.4 Discussion

The early morning hours are arguably the busiest time of day in Edogawa Care. The two staff on night shift, later partially supported by their colleague from the early day shift, need to get the floor's 50 or so residents out of bed, help them get dressed and go to the toilet, pick them up there again later on, and take them to the dayroom or, in some cases, back to bed for a few more minutes of rest. In between, they arrange things in the rooms, collect full and empty vessels, run for nappies and pads, attend to nurse calls, look after the residents in the washing section, serve tea in the dayroom, take the residents' vital signs, and talk.

This chapter has identified three recurring phenomena that show how this 'busy-ness' surfaces in the care workers' interactions with the residents. The first one is overlaps between turns, which have been explored in section 7.1. We have started with a few intentionally non-applicable cases, presented in order to clarify that overlaps can arise for a great number of reasons, of which only a minority relate to interactional tempo differences. The relevant cases, as we have seen in the later part of the section, are products of a 'rear-end collision' of two turns from different sequential stages. Where a resident's second pair part overlaps with a care worker's sequence closing third or new first pair part, the care worker is a whole turn 'ahead' of the resident in the interactional run.

In connection with the findings made in the analysis of the openings, in chapter 5, it is tempting to speculate on a possible relationship between a care worker's unwillingness to wait for a resident's second pair part, and the fact that so many opening greetings remain unanswered. Maybe the residents were just not quick enough to produce their reply to a greeting before a care worker would move the interaction on to the next stage.

Section 7.2 has taken a closer look at the interactional mechanics of multiple sayings. We have seen that such within-turn repetitions in the data fulfil two apparently opposite yet closely related functions. Repetitions of lexical items that designate parts of a resident's body or things to be 'attached' to it work as control acts intended to make a resident do something with these items. A closer verbal specification of the requested action is not given, but we can expect a large assortment of non-verbal devices such as gaze and gestures to go with these grammatically rudimentary instructions. The same holds for within-turn repetitions of deictic expressions that 'point' at a given direction a resident is requested to follow.

A second type of multiple saying is what with reference to Posenau (2014) I have referred to as 'brakes'. Such repetitions of warnings and other 'don't' directions are used by the care workers to halt a resident's current or imminent action. The analysis has shown that this type of multiple saying occurs both in such cases where a safety risk is involved (sitting down when there is nothing to sit on) and where it is not (produce this hand rather than that).

Thus multiple sayings in the data work towards either accelerating or decelerating a resident's action. What they have in common is that the care workers use both types in an attempt to control a resident's movements by adjusting the latter's tempo to their own tempo. This may also be a factor in accounting for the differing numbers of repeats. As I have hypothesised, there is some likeliness that a care worker's final repeat largely coincides with a resident's execution (or abortion) of the action the multiple saying refers to.

The third part of the analysis has focused on repetitions that occur as full turn units. Somewhat casually referred to in the previous chapters as 'prodding', this phenomenon describes the care workers' frequent attempts to 'pursue a response' (Pomerantz 1984b, Bolden et al. 2012) to a standing first pair part by offering a subsequent version of it. This produces a first non-uptake loop, which may be repeated as many times as necessary for a resident to deliver the required second pair part. The overall impression that arises is that while the care workers try to speed up things through reducing the space between turns, the residents do what they can to slow things down by broadening it.

With regard to this broadening of turn space, one thing we have only peripherally dealt with so far is that pauses are commonly seen as indicators of a dispreferred action (Pomerantz 1984a). We come back here to the initial observation by Davidson (1984) that a subsequent version of an offer, request, or similar type of first pair part is commonly delivered after a pause, and that this pause can be taken as a sign of hesitation or non-acceptance by the other speaker. An example from a care setting is presented in a study by Finlay and colleagues (2008), who analyse how two residents in a facility for people with intellectual disabilities refuse to cooperate in a task, and how the staff members work around these refusals. Both non-uptakes (on the part of the residents) and subsequent versions (by the staff) play an important part in these negotiations. If we apply this line of thought to the present data, this provides us with an alternative reason for the time gaps that frequently open up after the care workers' first pair parts. Rather than simply preferring to do things at a slower pace, a withheld reaction to a care worker's 'suggestion' about getting up or related actions may point, in at least some of the cases (e.g., excerpts 7.6 and 7.7), to a resident's general unwillingness to start the day at such an early hour.

It is hard to not see the numerous connections between the three phenomena discussed in this chapter. The special type of overlaps dealt with in section 7.1 is in fact a mirror image of the subsequent versions from section 7.3. Where the former is a case of 'more than one at a time', the latter is a device to deal with the opposite problem of 'fewer than one at a time' (Schegloff 2000: 2). The intention in both cases is to shrink the space between turns, or what Street and Buller (1988: 68) have referred to as 'response latency'. The result is a turn mismatch that bears uncanny similarities with exchanges in slightly time-lagged communication settings such as teleconferencing (see, e.g., Ruhleder and Jordan 2001). The main difference is that in the present data, the time lag is not a result of a technical transmission problem, but is entirely 'man-made'. A very similar pattern of turn mismatch has been observed in interactions between native and non-native speakers (Nakayama 2003: 203–204).

The most important (and most obvious) point that the multiple sayings from section 7.2 and the subsequent versions discussed in section 7.3 have in common is that both use the dynamics of repetition (Tannen 1987, Ishikawa 1991) to call for a resident's quick reaction. A major difference is that within-turn repeats seem to call for delivery of a physical action ('do/halt this'), while repetitions of whole turns call for a verbal one ('deliver required SPP'). Another parallel is that in both cases, there is some internal mechanism that makes repetitions speed themselves up. The acceleration that occurs on the word level in multiple sayings like *chie chechejeje* (excerpt 7.5) closely corresponds to the increasingly diminished length of turns and pauses that are commonly observed in subsequent versions.

What all three phenomena share is that they do not necessarily result in a quicker performance of the tasks – and can in fact have quite the opposite effect. With respect to overlaps, we have seen how the premature delivery of a sequence closing third fails to close the sequence as intended when, as in excerpt 7.3, it is produced in overlap with the resident's second pair part. This requires the resident to reconfirm her previous confirmation in an additional, fourth turn after the care worker's (non-)sequence closing third.

Regarding multiple sayings, we have seen that such within-turn repetitions transmit a considerable degree of urgency about a requested action, while not necessarily specifying that action itself in a sufficient way. For instance, as shown in the 'brake' example presented in excerpt 7.5, the care worker's unilateral rejection of a current action at first seems to leave the resident very much at a loss what to do. As also observed in Sassen's (2005) air traffic study, the multiple saying here takes on qualities of an expressive rather than a directive. Though perhaps the most intuitive way of giving directions when in a hurry, it may be more effective to choose a morphosyntactically more complex and semantically more specific format to communicate the requested action.

The counterproductive effect of interactional hurriedness becomes most salient in subsequent versions. Recall that what they are intended to do is accelerate a resident's delivery of a second pair part that a care worker regards as 'officially absent' (Schegloff 1968: 1088). However, in a sizeable number of cases, the second pair part actually was delivered, as in the example presented in excerpt 7.8, but went unnoticed by the busy care worker. This results in a long chain of subsequent versions without uptake, like a nervous driver who keeps hitting the gas out of gear.

That the production of hurriedness does not necessarily translate into quicker task performance has been observed in earlier studies in healthcare contexts, too. With respect to overlaps, Menz and Al-Roubaie (2008: 661) in their research on Austrian doctor–patient communication (see section 7.1) find that a doctor's interruptions 'performed in order to shorten a discussion will rather extend it!' A quite drastic example is presented by Staples (2015: 103–104), who shows how a nurse in a US hospital setting misses essential information due to her hurried delivery of questions without hearing what the patient has to say in reply.

Conversely, nurses interviewed by Chan et al. (2011: 1175) in a study on hospital communication in Hong Kong explicitly recognise 'the inherent value of chit-chat' during the care procedures, holding that it does not result in time loss but in fact helps to save time. Similarly, Heinemann (2009a) in her research on communication in a Danish home help setting observes how a detour of humour and joking prior to an upcoming care task in effect contributes to a quicker performance of that task.

While these are interesting findings that deserve follow-up research, I think that the question of how much a less hurried interactional style can actually contribute to a quicker performance of the care tasks should not get us on the wrong track. Apart from the fact that the actual amount of time to be 'saved' would add up to no more than a few seconds per interaction, the main reason for a slower way of doing things, in my view, should be that it would relate to a more symmetrical way of communication between caregiver and care recipient, and hence to a better way of providing and receiving care. As Jansson and Plejert (2014: 55) emphasise in their study on dementia care in Sweden, what really matters is 'not time-savings but greater rapport and interpersonal harmony'.

What is all this hurry for in the first place? When addressing this question to the care workers in our final study session, they explained that they wanted some leeway (*yoyū*) before breakfast, which is served at 7:30. They specified that a resident might feel sick or want to go to the toilet once more, so they needed time for such eventualities to be addressed. Also, they found it easier to watch over (*mimamoru*) the residents when they were assembled in the dayroom. To this end, they were normally trying to have most residents at their table about an hour (!) in advance of breakfast time.

While these first-hand views by the participants naturally deserve to be respected, there may be a couple of other reasons involved in the care workers' hurried interaction style. This is a point we will return to in the concluding chapter.

8 Conclusions

Having examined the data with respect to, in reverse order of appearance, the interactional tempo, the back and forth of task talk and non-task talk, the organisation of openings and closings, and the occurrence of honorifics, we now come back to the overall research question that has motivated this study and guided us through the analysis: What are the basic characteristics of care communication – as we find them in staff–resident interactions during the morning care procedures in Edogawa Care? The qualification after the dash is important, as it reminds us that we have in fact been studying only one specific type of interaction, in one specific type of setting. Obviously, generalisations are feasible only up to a certain point.

In summary, the previous chapters have shown that the type of communication explored in this book is characterised by three major attributes: It is

(1) task-focused,
(2) asymmetrical, and
(3) done in a hurry.

After briefly reviewing each of the three points, we will turn to two larger sociolinguistic topics that have been looming in the background throughout the analysis, and that can now be addressed in a more coherent manner. The chapter closes with a few personal observations regarding the importance of communication in institutional eldercare.

8.1 Main characteristics of care communication

In line with many observations from previous studies, one major characteristic of communication in Edogawa Care is the task-orientedness of the interactions. This becomes manifest in a great variety of features, including: a high number of exchanges without any non-task related talk; the regular occurrence of silences during the task work; a large variety of directives and inquiries about running or impending care tasks; the common use of material such as heave-hoes and transition markers to prepare, perform, and acknowledge physical actions; a mutual understanding among the participants that task talk overrules non-task talk; and the swift closing of an exchange once the last task has been completed. All of this leaves little doubt that it is the tasks that bring the participants together, not the talk.

Two reservations are in order here. First, non-task talk can and does occur. As we have seen in chapter 6, the participants frequently fill in the time spent working on the tasks to discuss matters other than the things they happen to be doing. This includes anything from prototypical 'small talk', such as short sequences about the weather or the time, to considerably 'big' stories that provide substantial insights into the storyteller's non-institutional life. A closer look at non-task talk has further revealed that it is not the sole responsibility of the care workers to proffer, allow, or withhold such sequences, but that the care recipients play an active part in making non-task talk happen – or not, if they prefer to do without.

The second point is that the attested focus on the tasks and the structural consequences this entails are by no means confined to interactions in eldercare contexts. As Goffman (1981: 133) reminds us, '[i]ndeed, there are a great number of work settings where informal talk is subordinated to the task at hand, the accommodation being not to another conversation but to the exigencies of work in progress'. Most of the talk produced in such settings, Goffman (1981: 143) continues, is 'coordinated task activity – not conversation'. A similar point was made by Fiehler (1980: 66), who holds that communication in such 'practically dominated activity contexts' mainly serves to organise ongoing activities. More recent research goes even further in questioning the 'logocentric' bias in analysing interactions and propagating a 'hierarchical primacy of embodied behavior over speech' in the management of joint activities in various contexts (Stevanovic and Monzoni 2016: 30).

Rather than making over-critical evaluations regarding the dominance of the tasks, we should acknowledge this as a general feature of talk in institutional settings. The interesting point is how the participants orient to this feature in interactions, thereby talking the institution into and – at times – out of being, as exemplified in section 6.3.

The second characteristic that shapes the interactions is the pronounced asymmetries between care workers and residents. As with the previous point, we should keep in mind that this is a feature of institutional interactions in general. However, as we have seen throughout all four chapters of the analysis, the 'total' nature of residential eldercare seems to further amplify the predominance of the institutional representatives.

No doubt the most obvious indication of how the care workers are 'in charge' during the morning care is the high frequency of control acts. The analysis in section 6.1.1 has shown that an overwhelming majority of all directives are made by the staff. We have also seen that, in many cases, this 'making someone do something' takes a markedly direct format, thus expressing a considerable degree of entitlement on the part of the care workers.

The staff's dominance is further reflected in address term usage, as discussed in chapter 4. Whereas most of the interactions contain at least one term of address used by the staff towards a resident, there are only a handful of cases in which a resident uses an address term towards the staff. One likely factor for this imbalance is access to knowledge: Residents simply may not know a care worker's name. On the other hand, we have also seen that the largest part of all address terms by the care workers are used as vocatives rather than in referential function, thus serving as a device for interactional control. If we subtract these 'summons items' from the corpus and focus only on referential usage, the number of address terms used by residents and staff is basically on par.

But asymmetries do not only surface in the occurrence of certain speech acts or lexical items. As a look at common sequence types has shown, they are written into the very structure of the exchanges. At the heart of this structure is a care worker's first pair part (of a greeting, a control act, an inquiry, etc.), which automatically assigns a reactive, second pair part role to the resident. Moreover, the care worker often repeats a first pair part to mark a resident's reply as missing. Where it is delivered, the care worker habitually acknowledges receipt with a sequence closing third. In other words, we have a nuclear (CW:FPP) (Res:SPP) structure, which is commonly extended into (CW:FPP) (CW:FPP^n) (Res:SPP) (CW:SCT), where n refers to the number of possible repeats.

Noteworthy about this structure is that it not only allocates a higher number of turns to the care worker. Even more important is that it provides for a pattern in which the care worker by default both opens and closes a sequence. Note that the same structural characteristic replicates itself on a larger level, in that it is also the care worker who habitually opens and closes an interaction as a whole. Seen in this light, it seems that care communication, or at least the task talk part of it, is more akin to interactions in formal (as opposed to informal) institutional settings than one might think (see section 2.2).

On the other hand, we have also come across various deviations from these patterns of asymmetry. For example, with respect to both openings and closings, we have seen how a reversal of the turn structure can temporarily put the resident in charge of the flow of events. Such cases, rare as they may be, serve to show that institutional asymmetry is no pre-given state, but an interactional product that the participants can refuse to deliver.

The third feature of communication in Edogawa Care is urgency. As in many other care settings, the interactions studied appear to be strongly 'constrained by time and task' (Davis and Pope 2010: 37). While this condition is commonly acknowledged in studies on care (e.g., Duffy et al. 2015), its interactional consequences have to my knowledge not been explored in more depth so far. The aim of chapter 7 has been to determine how the state of being hurried manifests itself in the data, thereby leaving its marks on some fundamental parts of the sequential structure.

To briefly summarise the main points, the data are characterised by a large number of overlaps that result from the clash of a 'delayed' second pair part by a resident with a subsequent 'new' turn by the care worker. In addition, the care workers commonly repeat turn-internal material or whole turns in order to accelerate a verbal or physical reaction by a resident. Somewhat ironically, the analysis has shown that this sort of interactional hurriedness does not always translate into quicker task performance, but can even have contrary effects.

Given that there is not that much to be gained from hurriedness per se, we now come back to the question why this interactional style occurs in the first place. Most insightful in this respect is a study conducted by Naitō (2006), which has been briefly described in the literature review in chapter 2. Naitō video-recorded resident–staff interactions during meal time in three Japanese care facilities for dementia patients. These recordings were subsequently shown to other care professionals, who were asked for comments. One thing they observed was that their featured colleagues frequently announced an upcoming action that was acknowledged by a resident only 'after the fact', that is, when the action itself had already been performed. Note that the underlying structure of this phenomenon, a mismatch between action and reaction, closely resembles the special type of overlaps described in section 7.1.

Naitō's experiment further enabled him to elicit a few revealing comments about the motivations for this type of behaviour. According to the expert viewers – as said, care professionals themselves – one of the likely reasons for the staff's hurriedness was the perceived necessity to constantly 'be doing' something, even when this was clearly not in line with the current needs or preferences of the care recipients. As Naitō (2006: 110) points out, this seems to relate to the idea that 'fussing around' (*komagoma to ugoku koto*) is generally considered a positive attribute of eldercare professionals. Considering the reverse side of this argument, this means that a care worker who attends to care recipients at a slower pace, intentionally or not, may easily be regarded as less capable of 'doing care' than her or his more busily working peers.

I would like to add a few remarks from my own experiences in institutional eldercare (see chapter 1). In the German home where I used to work, the (daytime) shifts on Saturdays and Sundays were normally staffed with fewer than the regular number of care workers, in order to assure that the fulltime staff could get at least each second weekend off. This meant that those who happened to be on a weekend shift would have more work to do than during the week. In effect though, I always had the impression that work on weekends was somewhat less exhausting and more easily done than on ordinary working days. The main reason for this, as I remember it, was that the lower number of staff on duty also provided an 'excuse' to work through the tasks more quickly, with less attention to interpersonal matters. A quick pace thus may also be a possible way to reduce the amount of 'emotional labour' (Hochschild 1983, Smith 2012, Erickson and Stacey 2013) involved in such a psychologically taxing job.

And yet there is a counter-perspective to this argument. Yumi Muguruma, a former Japanese university professor who quit her job to become a professional care worker, in 2012 published a critically acclaimed self-ethnography about her personal experiences in institutional eldercare. She focuses particularly on the many life stories she was told by the people she was looking after, which to her as a trained ethnographer constitute a true 'treasure trove' (*hōko*) of lived memories. This leads her to describe the new job in a very positive and uncommonly optimistic way throughout the book. The general tone temporarily changes when, in the closing chapter, she describes how, due to a transfer to a different section, she now finds herself working under constant time pressure and without being able to make room for listening to the residents' stories. According to her account, this entailed some serious emotional stress, and significantly lowered her work satisfaction. These very personal insights, which I am happy to acknowledge, suggest that there is something in it for both sides if sufficient time can be taken to 'care'.

8.2   Doing gender, doing care

One big topic that has kept popping up throughout the analysis is gender. To start with the simple part, the analysis of the data has frequently shown a relatively straightforward effect of the participants' biological sex on the way they speak or are spoken to. In chapter 4, for instance, we have seen that the beautified form *o-toire* is almost exclusively used by female speakers. The analysis of terms of address has revealed that female residents tend to be called by their first name more often than their male peers. With respect to how the residents address the care workers, I have discussed one special case where a male resident uses the hypercoristic -*chan* address towards a female staff member (who, as mentioned, happened to be the station nurse). Conversely, the data do not contain any instances of the -*kun* address, which would be the closest corresponding male version of -*chan*. These examples illustrate how persisting gender inequalities in society come to be reflected in language usage, a problem that has stimulated much research ever since Robin Lakoff's (1975) seminal publication on the topic.

On the other hand, it is now common sense in sociolinguistics and related fields that gender is anything but a stable variable. Rather than a fixed binary distinction that produces linguistic output 'off the peg', gender has come to be considered a resource that speakers use to perform diverse and alternating identities through their linguistic choices. This makes them 'active producers rather than passive reproducers of gendered behaviour' (Cameron 1997: 50). According to this view, as Coates (2004: vi) summarises, 'gender is no longer seen as a given but rather as something that we "do"'.

That the participants in our study are doing this in different ways, and to differing extents, can best be understood from the dramatic dissimilarities in the speech of the two male care workers. The transcripts juxtaposed in section 4.2.2 (see excerpts 4.2 and 4.3) have demonstrated that the speech of Sm1 has some clear characteristics of what is normally associated with the 'toughness' of male speech, whereas Sm2 uses a softer, stereotypically more female register. The analysis of the two excerpts has also shown that the difference is by no means confined to the use and non-use of the formal style, but becomes manifest in a variety of discursive features.

To back up this point with more evidence from other examples discussed, we may add that it is Sm1 who in excerpt 5.7 raises the 'getting up' issue before even greeting the resident, just as it is him who uses a multiple saying to make the resident produce the 'right' hand in excerpt 7.5. By contrast, Sm2 empathically listens to the resident's sewing machine story (excerpts 6.12 and 6.13) and apologises for not having learned to sew himself (excerpt 6.14).

Focusing on Sm1, a look at the whole sample shows that there are other stereotypically male characteristics he habitually equips his speech with. One is his exclusive use of the first person pronoun *ore*, as opposed to Sm2, who uses both *ore* and the 'less-manly' *boku* (SturtzSreetharan 2009: 262). It is also Sm1 who gives the most straightforward directives of all care workers, including forms such as *owattara osun da yo:* 'When finished you push' (#101'51) and *hitori de yattcha dame da yo:* 'Don't you do this by yourself' (#57'272). On the phonological level, his speech is marked by a habitual vowel coalescence of /ai/ into /ee/, as in *okiru ka okinee ka kiiterun da ke do* 'If you're getting up or not's what I'm asking' (#105'37), a feature commonly classified as 'strongly masculine' (e.g., Okamoto 1995, 2016). None of his colleagues ever use this pronunciation in the data.

The interesting point is that, on the other hand, these characteristics of Sm1's speech combine with a number of traits normally considered prototypical parts of female language. Thus he frequently produces sentences with a deleted copula verb before a sentence-final particle, as in *san nin de yaru wake yo* 'We work in threes' (#46'23). He also shows a preference for marking his questions with the particle *no*, like in *asoo na no?* 'Oh really?' (#99'49) or *moo chotto otchatte ii no?* 'Can I fold this up a little more?' (#107'85). And even the excerpt discussed in section 4.2.2 contains a rather feminine sentence-final form, the pairing of *no* and *ne* in his summarising observation *nemureta no ne* 'So you could sleep then' (see excerpt 4.2). While these features all can and do occur in male speech, too, it is interesting to note that our second male care worker, Sm2, never uses any of them. These tendencies may also serve to explain why it is that Sm1, rather than Sm2, produces the only three instances of beautified *o-toire* in male speech, which seemed somewhat hard to account for when first discussed in section 4.3.3.

The gender ambiguity of Sm1's speech becomes perhaps most salient in a nurse call sequence at the very peak of one day's morning care activities. In it, he tells the resident at the other end of the line that the care workers are very busy right now because everyone is getting up and, therefore, *natte mo shoo ga nee no yo* 'It's no use however much you ring' (#47'44). While the pronunciation of the negation marker *nai* as *nee* is clearly marked for stereotypically male speech, the combination of the two sentence-final particles *no* and *yo* is a common characteristic of female speech (e.g., Ide and Yoshida 1999, Inoue 2006: 242, 259, SturtzSreetharan 2009). This creates a rather complex hybrid of 'female grammar' delivered in a male voice.

These observations must be contextualised within the special type of setting under observation. Work in care and nursing professions, in Japan as elsewhere, is commonly considered to be 'women's work' (P. Smith 1992, Williams 1993, Thimm 1997). Previous studies have identified various strategies of how men in such 'non-traditional occupations' tend to reconcile their professional identities with the normative gender mismatch they face (Heikes 1991, Lupton 2000, Cross and Bagilhole 2002, Simpson 2004).

One of the few studies that deal with the linguistic characteristics of such situations is McDowell (2015a, 2015b). Her audio-recordings of three male nurses in a Northern Irish hospital reveal that the participants' interactional style embraces a variety of properties commonly associated with women's speech, including a large number of mitigation devices, gossiping, and shared humour. Interestingly, this was not quite in line with the participants' self-perceptions, as McDowell found out in semi-structured interviews. The male nurses in her study went out of their way to emphasise the difference of their speech with that of their female co-workers, maintaining that 'they could not conform to feminine discourse as this would conflict with their masculine identity' (McDowell 2015b: 373). McDowell's analysis of their actual speech output seems to tell a different story.

Coming back to the two male care workers in the present study, we are now in a better position to appreciate how the feminised work environment may come to bear on their way of speaking. In the case of Sm2, this becomes most obvious in his non-assertive interactional style, of which his frequent use of formal speech – more frequent than any of his female colleagues, as the analysis in section 4.2.1 has revealed – is but one example. As for Sm1, an endless number of instances could be added to demonstrate that his communicative behaviour on first look is as prototypically male as can be. Yet, as we have just seen, his speech shows some undeniable traces of what is commonly characterised as Japanese women's language, suggesting that he, too, is negotiating and readjusting his male identity in this prototypically female occupational setting.

8.3   Politeness and impoliteness

A second noisy background topic, and one closely linked to language and gender in fact, is politeness. As specified in the introductory part of chapter 4, I have intentionally kept the analysis there focused on honorifics, anticipating that it would be all but impossible to deal with a topic as complex as politeness within the confines of a single chapter. In view of the study's broader research interest, this approach has certainly had its merits. Among other things, it has allowed us to see that a casual, almost family-like way of speech is the default mode in Edogawa Care, and that this is most likely a result of the intimate care actions the participants are required to perform with one another. While I do think this is a worthwhile finding in its own right, the larger topic of politeness has remained an elephant in the room. It is time to deal with this oversized mammal now.

First off, it is clear but perhaps worth restating that honorifics are but a small and purely 'symptomatic' aspect of politeness. Following Holmes (2012: 208), politeness can be conceptualised as 'discursively strategic interaction, i.e. linguistic devices perceived as having been used in order to maintain harmonious relations and avoid conflict with others'. This being the case, politeness is not simply manifested in certain speech forms per se, but needs to be approached as a discursive phenomenon that revolves around the participants' face needs and how their talk is oriented to this (e.g., Kasper 2006, Geyer 2008a).

With respect to the care data, this means that we should not be looking for politeness in the mere use of address terms, formal speech, beautification prefixes, and other things we have studied in chapter 4. Rather, politeness becomes relevant in the organisation of openings and closings (chapter 5), different ways of communicating care tasks and care non-related matters (chapter 6), and, of course, the negotiation of tempo differences (chapter 7). Analysing these phenomena, we have frequently bumped into issues that directly relate to the participants' face needs and how they are addressed, or not, in interaction.

Relevant topics include how to meet and un-meet in an efficient but mutually agreed way, how to attend to the other person's storytelling and get one's own stories told, how to insert pieces of task talk into these stories in a minimally intrusive way, and how to break out of one's predefined institutional roles through the use of humour and verbal play. Countless instances in the data serve to show that the participants are well aware of each other's face needs, and do what they can to reconcile them with the ongoing task work. This includes both whole speech acts like greetings, apologies, and expressions of gratitude, and micro devices such as backchannelling, mitigation, and laughter, used by the participants on a moment-by-moment basis to show they 'care' for each other.

On the other hand, the analysis has also come across quite a number of issues that would fall into the realm of impoliteness, a topic of growing interest in recent politeness research (e.g., Bousfield and Locher 2008, Culpeper 2011). Though there is as yet no unified definition of the concept, most researchers minimally agree that impoliteness relates to acts of intended or accidental disregard of another's face needs. Phenomena of likely relevance from the present study are looming conflicts with respect to the issue of getting up, overly directive control acts in task talk, rejection of non-task talk initiations, and openly displayed impatience while waiting for pending second pair parts, to name but a few.

Impoliteness also becomes a relevant issue with respect to the topic of patronising talk (see section 2.2). In her seminal study on care communication in Wales, Grainger (1993a) draws a direct connection between impoliteness and infantilisation. She observes that the elderly patients in her data are often 'assigned a child-like role and therefore are not expected to have the same face wants as adults'. Some care workers in her data appeared to 'assume that dependency also implies a loss of normal adult politeness conventions' (Grainger 1993a: 249). Sachweh (2000: 178) makes a similar point in her German study, which includes a long list of face threatening acts that show the staff's 'ambivalent attitudes regarding the residents' adult status'. Various other examples of 'practices that threatened residents' adult identities' are given by Ryvicker (2009: 23) in an ethnographic study in two US nursing homes.

Indeed, a closer look at previous research on interactions between parents and children reveals some rather uncanny similarities to what we have observed in the present study. For instance, Craven and Potter (2010: 423), who examined dinner table interactions in the UK, found that many of the parents' directives in their data qualify as 'telling rather than asking', similar to the relatively straightforward way in which the majority of the control acts in the present study are formulated. In a joint research project from Sweden and the US, Goodwin and Cekaite (2013: 129, 133) further observe the regular use of hortative forms and a specific 'boundary marker + noun phrase' directive, both of which frequently occur in my sample, too (see section 6.1.1).

Another relevant feature is subsequent versions. Craven and Potter (2010: 431) state that in their parent–child data, 'non-compliance with directives recurrently leads to upgraded (more entitled and less contingent) repeat directives'. They also observe that these repetitions are frequently shorter than the original version, as though to express 'an increased sense of urgency' (Craven and Potter 2010: 433). Though not predominantly directives, the subsequent versions explored in section 7.3 seem to have just that function.

Repetition has also been identified as an important strategy in Japanese caregiver–child interaction. For instance, Burdelski (2010: 1610) presents a sequence in which a teacher in a day care centre produces three subsequent versions to make a child deliver a requested 'thank you' turn. Similar observations have been made in parent–child interaction. Studies by Clancy (1986), Kobayashi (2001), and Endo and Takada (2016) discuss various cases in which parents use repetitions and upgrades to make their child follow a requested course of action, in a very similar way to what we have observed in chapter 7.

As these examples show, a great number of the interactional peculiarities in the eldercare data seem to be close replicates of characteristic parent–child talk, with the care worker adopting the parent role and the resident that of the child. It is particularly this disregard of a resident's adulthood – combined with the inherent element of control – that makes many of the observed phenomena qualify as instances of impoliteness.

One likely conclusion that evolves from the discussion is that, paradoxically, it now almost looks as though the chapter on honorifics has had less to do with the topic of politeness than the three subsequent chapters. Contrarily, various parts of the analysis have shown how honorifics fulfil functions that are not primarily related to the problems discussed in chapter 4. Regarding terms of address, for instance, rather than variation between first name and last name, what seems to matter most is their predominant use by the care workers as summons items to assure a resident's attention. Conversely, the virtual non-occurrence of fictively used kinship terms, commendable as it is, does not mean that patronising talk is not an issue in Edogawa Care.

A similar observation applies to the use of addressee honorifics. As we have seen, speech style choice fulfils a number of vital functions only peripherally related to face issues. For instance, the analysis in chapter 6 has shown that alternations between formal and plain speech in many cases coincide with shifts between task talk and non-task talk. In addition, as chapter 7 has revealed, downgrading from formal to plain is a common phenomenon in subsequent versions, where it serves to mark the absence of a pending second pair part. To some extent, the same may even hold for the use and non-use of beautification prefixes, as excerpt 4.7 has suggested. While all of these phenomena are not entirely unrelated to the topic of politeness, their primary function is to organise the interactional flow. In sum, then, it is safe to say that honorifics are at least as important for structuring the discourse as they are for managing interpersonal relationships.

8.4 Who cares?

Little things make a difference. This is one of the main messages in Pam Smith's (1992) now classic *The emotional labour of nursing*, and it seemed more valid than ever when the second edition of the book appeared in 2012. Drawing on years of experience in nursing education, Smith cites many of these 'little things' as highly important for the quality of care, including remembering anniversaries, making sure patients have clean glasses, and letting them dress in their own clothes. While in the eyes of many a staff member, these may seem mere 'trivialities' (Persson and Wästerfors 2009), desirable but beyond the expectable, Smith (2012: 3) emphasises that their absence is in fact 'stark evidence of the lack of care'.

Language is one of these little things, as Posenau (2013) is anxious to point out in a recent article for a German journal on care work. And yet the overall importance of communication in institutional eldercare is by no means as obvious to care professionals as it may be to the linguist or social scientist. Looking back to the very beginning of this project, I remember how I had a hard time explaining to the then director of Edogawa Care, a trained physician specialised in neurosurgery, what exactly my research was all about. Even though he was amazingly cooperative from the start, he made no bones about admitting that he could not quite get the purpose of this whole project, given that it was 'only about how people talk' (*shabetteru dake*).

I was in for a couple of more such moments of disenchantment later on, during the study sessions with the care workers. While I did receive a lot of positive feedback, particularly in the form of acknowledgements that mere listening to their own speech substantially raised their consciousness about the importance of language at work, they had many issues they considered more urgent than talk. I remember particularly well one instance where I presented with some enthusiasm my 'discovery' regarding the interactional significance of *o-toire* 'toilet'(beautified) as opposed to *toire* (non-beautified). Their less enthusiastic reaction told me this: They could not care less.

Needless to say, both the director and the care workers have a point. It is hard to deny that there are bigger issues in Japanese eldercare than just 'how people talk'. How can we make sure a growing number of old people will get the care they need? How much is Japanese society willing to pay for this? What can be done to improve the working conditions for care professionals and counter the high turnover rate in this job? And what role in current and future welfare schemes is there to play for a 'non-native' workforce, including both foreign care workers and robots? Aren't these the real issues?

I agree. Given current and projected demographic trends, Japan's quickly ageing society is facing enormous structural problems with respect to both quality and quantity of eldercare. The nature of care communication as I have sketched it in this study – its heavy focus on task work, its asymmetries, its hurriedness – in many ways is but a product of these background conditions. Yet, on the other hand, it is my conviction – as a linguist, one-time care worker, and prospective care recipient some years down the line – that language does matter. When it comes to the micro-level of human interaction, talk is one of the most immediate ways to show one 'cares'. And while this book does not present any fit-all models for care communication, it hopefully serves to show how the little things can make a difference in the various ways people care for each other as they try to make a home in an unlikely place.

References

Akashi, Junichi. 2014. New aspects of Japan's immigration policies: Is population decline opening the doors? *Contemporary Japan* 26(2). 175–196. http://www.tandfonline.com/doi/abs/10.1515/cj-2014-0009 (accessed 24 January 2017).

Akiya, Naonori. 2008. Kōreisha kaigo shisetsu ni miru kaiwa kōzō: nichijō seikatsu ni okeru ji/ta kaiwa bunseki [Conversational structure in an eldercare facility: A conversation analysis of self/other in everyday life]. *Hoken iryō shakaigaku ronbunshū* 19(2). 56–67. http://ci.nii.ac.jp/naid/110009845359 (accessed 31 August 2016).

Akiya, Naonori, Rie Kawashima & Keiichi Yamazaki. 2009b. Kea bamen ni okeru sanyo chii no haibun: hanashite ni naru koto to ukete ni naru koto [Allocation of participant status in care settings: Becoming speaker and becoming recipient]. *Ninchi kagaku* 16(1). 78–90.

Akiya, Naonori, Hitoshi Niwa, Yoshinori Kuno & Keiichi Yamazaki. 2006. Fukushi robotto kaihatsu no tame no irai purosesu ni kan suru kihonteki kōsatsu [Basic considerations about the requesting process for the development of a welfare robot]. *Fukushi jōhō kōgaku* 105(684). 35–40.

Akiya, Naonori, Hitoshi Niwa, Mai Okada, Keiichi Yamazaki, Yoshinori Kobayashi, Yoshinori Kuno & Akiko Yamazaki. 2009a. Kōreisha kaigo shisetsu ni okeru komyunikēshon channeru kakuritsu katei no bunseki to shien shisutemu no teian [Analysis of the setup process of a communication channel and proposal for a support system in an eldercare facility]. *Jōhō shori gakkai ronbunshū* 50(1). 302–313. http://id.nii.ac.jp/1001/00009335/ (accessed 31 August 2016).

Akiya, Naonori, Hitoshi Niwa, Hisao Tsubota, Sachie Tsuruta, Hideaki Kuzuoka, Yoshinori Kuno & Keiichi Yamazaki. 2007. Kaigo robotto kaihatsu ni muketa kōreisha kaigo shisetsu ni okeru sōgo kōi no shakaigakuteki bunseki [A sociological analysis of interaction for care robot development in an eldercare facility]. *Denshi jōhō tsūshin gakkai ronbunshi* D, *Jōhō/shisutemu* J90-D(3). 798–807.

Akiya, Naonori, Keiichi Yamazaki, Kouji Mitsuhashi & Yoshinori Kuno. 2008. Kōreisha kaigo shisetsu ni okeru irai kōi no sōgo kōi bunseki [Interactional analysis of request behaviour in an eldercare facility]. *Jōhō shori gakkai dai 70 kai zenkoku taikai*. 101–102. http://id.nii.ac.jp/1001/00138384/ (accessed 31 August 2016).

Akizuki, Kōtarō. 2015. 'Gozaru' no gengogaku [The linguistics of *gozaru*]. *Shōkei gakuin daigaku kiyō* 69. 53–66. http://ci.nii.ac.jp/naid/110009954371 (accessed 31 August 2016).

Amada, Josuke. 1997. Shisetsu nyūsho chihōsei rōjin no robī ni okeru sōgo sayō tokusei ni kan suru kenkyū [Research on the characteristics of lobby interaction between institutionalised dementia patients]. *Rōnen shakai kagaku* 19(1). 39–47.

Amada, Josuke. 1999. 'Chihōsei rōjin' ni okeru, arui wa 'chihōsei rōjin' o meguru sōgo sayō no shosō [Interpretations of social interaction of, or around, 'demented elders']. *Shakai fukushigaku* 40(1). 209–233.

Angles, Jeffrey, Ayumi Nagatomi & Mineharu Nakayama. 2000. Japanese responses *hai*, *ee*, and *un*: Yes, no, and beyond. *Language and Communication* 20. 55–86.

Antaki, Charles & Rebecca J. Crompton. 2015. Conversational practices promoting a discourse of agency for adults with intellectual disabilities. *Discourse & Society* 26(6). 645–661.

Antaki, Charles, W. Mick L. Finlay, Chris Walton & Joe Sempik. 2016. Communicative practices in staff support of adults with intellectual disabilities. In J.N. Lester & M. O'Reilly (eds.), *The Palgrave handbook of adult mental health*, 613–632. Houndmills: Palgrave Macmillan.

Antaki, Charles & Alexandra Kent. 2012. Telling people what to do (and, sometimes, why): Contingency, entitlement and explanation in staff requests to adults with intellectual impairments. *Journal of Pragmatics* 44(6/7). 876–889.

Aoki, Mizuho. 2016. Nursing care workers hard to find but in demand in aging Japan. *Japan Times*, 26 June. http://www.japantimes.co.jp/news/2016/06/27/reference/nursing-care-workers-hard-to-find-but-in-demand-in-aging-japan/#.V3EnS_l9601 (accessed 31 August 2016).

Aoyama, Katsura. 2002. Request strategies at a Japanese workplace. In A. Bell, J. Shoemaker & G. Sibley (eds.), *Selected papers from the third college-wide conference for students in languages, linguistics and literature 1999*, 3–11. Honolulu: Second Language Teaching & Curriculum Center, University of Hawaii at Manoa.

Arminen, Ikka. 2005. *Institutional interaction: Studies of talk at work*. Aldershot & Burlington: Ashgate.

Armstrong-Esther, C.A., K.D. Browne & J.G. McAfee. 1994. Elderly patients: Still clean and sitting quietly. *Journal of Advanced Nursing* 19(2). 264–271.

Aronsson, Karin & Asta Cekaite. 2011. Activity contracts and directives in everyday family politics. *Discourse & Society* 22(2). 137–154.

Aronsson, Karin & Bengt Rundström. 1989. Cats, dogs and sweets in the clinical negotiation of reality: On politeness and coherence in pediatric discourse. *Language in Society* 18(4). 483–504.

Asahi Shimbun. 2015. 2030 nen robotto to watashi [Robots and me 2030], 31 March, p. 11.

Atkinson, John M. & John Heritage (eds.). 1984. *Structures of social action*. Cambridge: Cambridge University Press.

Backhaus, Peter. 2008. Coming to terms with age: Some linguistic consequences of population ageing. In F. Coulmas, H. Conrad, A. Schad-Seifert & G. Vogt (eds.), *The demographic challenge: A handbook about Japan*, 455–471. Leiden & Boston: Brill.

Backhaus, Peter. 2009. Politeness in institutional elderly care in Japan: A cross-cultural comparison. *Journal of Politeness Research* 5(1). 53–71.

Backhaus, Peter. 2010. Time to get up: Compliance-gaining in a Japanese eldercare facility. *Journal of Asian Pacific Communication* 20(1). 69–89.

Backhaus, Peter. 2011. 'Me nurse, you resident': Institutional role-play in a Japanese caring facility. In P. Backhaus (ed.), *Communication in elderly care: Cross-cultural perspectives*, 129–144. London & New York: Continuum.

Backhaus, Peter. 2016. Ubiquitous and conveniently vague: Let's look at -ō and -shō. *Japan Times*, 11 April. http://www.japantimes.co.jp/life/2016/04/11/language/ubiquitous-conveniently-vague-lets-look-o-sho/#.Vyy2bISLTIV (accessed 31 August 2016).

Bailey, Benjamin. 2008. Interactional sociolinguistics. In W. Donsbach (ed.), *The international encyclopedia of communication*, 2314–2318. New York: Blackwell.

Bangerter, Adrian & Herbert H. Clark. 2003. Navigating joint projects with dialogue. *Cognitive Science* 27(2). 195–225.

Barke, Andrew. 2010. Manipulating honorifics in the construction of social identities in Japanese television drama. *Journal of Sociolinguistics* 14(4). 456–476.

Barke, Andrew. 2011. Situated (im)politeness and the use of addressee honorifics in Japanese television dramas. In B.L. Davies, M. Haugh & A.J. Merrison (eds.), *Situated politeness*, 111–128. London & New York: Continuum.

Bataller, Rebecca. 2015. Pragmatic variation in the performance of requests: A comparative study of service encounters in Valencia and Granada (Spain). In María de la O Hernández-López & Lucía Fernández-Amaya (eds.), *A multidisciplinary approach to service encounters*, 113–137. Leiden & Boston: Brill.

Beach, Wayne A. 1995. Preserving and constraining options: 'Okays' and official priorities in medical interviews. In J.H. Morris & R.J. Chenail (eds.), *The talk of the clinic: Explorations in the analysis of medical and therapeutic discourse*, 259–289. Hillsdale: Erlbaum.

Beck, Christina S. & Sandra L. Ragan. 1995. Negotiating relational and medical talk: Frame shifts in the gynecologic exam. *Journal of Language and Social Psychology* 11(1). 47–61.

Becker, Alton L. 1984. The linguistics of particularity: Interpreting superordination in a Javanese text. In C. Brugman & M. Macaulay (eds.), *Proceedings of the tenth annual meeting of the Berkeley Linguistics Society*, 425–436. Berkeley: University of California Press.

Beckman, Howard B. & Richard M. Frankel. 1984. The effect of physician behavior on the collection of data. *Annals of Internal Medicine* 101(5). 692–696.

Belz, Julie A. & Celeste Kinginger. 2003. Discourse options and the development of pragmatic competence by classroom learners of German: The case of address forms. *Language Learning* 53(4). 591–647.

Berenz, Norine. 2001. Interactional sociolinguistic research methods. In R. Mesthrie (ed.), *Concise encyclopedia of sociolinguistics*, 784–787. Oxford: Elsevier.

Bethel, Diana Lynn. 1992a. Life on Obasuteyama, or, inside a Japanese institution for the elderly. In T.S. Lebra (ed.), *Japanese social organization*, 109–134. Honolulu: University of Hawaii Press.

Bethel, Diana Lynn. 1992b. Alienation and reconnection in a home for the elderly. In J.J. Tobin (ed.), *Re-made in Japan: Everyday life and consumer taste in a changing society*, 126–142. New Haven: Yale University Press.

Bilmes, Jack. 1997. Being interrupted. *Language in Society* 26(4). 507–531.

Blum-Kulka, Shoshana, Juliane House & Gabriele Kasper (eds.). 1989. *Cross-cultural pragmatics: Requests and apologies*. Norwood: Ablex.

Bolden, Galina B., Jenny Mandelbaum & Sue Wilkinson. 2012. Pursuing a response by repairing an indexical reference. *Research on Language and Social Interaction* 45(2). 137–155.

Bousfield, Derek & Miriam A. Locher (eds.). 2008. *Impoliteness in language: Studies on its interplay with power in theory and practice*. Berlin & New York: De Gruyter.

Braun, Friederike. 1988. *Terms of address: Problems of patterns and usage in various languages and cultures*. Berlin: Mouton de Gruyter.

Brown, Penelope & Stephen C. Levinson. 1987. *Politeness: Some universals in language usage*. Cambridge: Cambridge University Press.

Brown, Roger & Marguerite Ford. 1961. Address in American English. *Journal of Abnormal Social Psychology* 62(2). 375–385.

Brown, Roger W. & Albert Gilman. 1960. The pronouns of power and solidarity. In T. Sebeok (ed.), *Style in language*, 253–276. Cambridge: MIT Press.

Bu, Yan. 2004. Koshō ni okeru poraitonesu shinri kōsatsu: shinzoku meishō no kyokōteki yōhō ni kan suru nichi/chū/eigo hikaku [Considerations on the politeness psychology of address terms: A comparison of the fictive use of kinship terms in Japanese, Chinese, and English]. *Shukutoku daigaku shakai gakubu kenkyū kiyō* 38. 313–328. http://ci.nii.ac.jp/naid/110004786406 (accessed 31 August 2016).

Bunkacho (Agency for Cultural Affairs). 2007. Keigo no shishin [Principles of polite language]. http://keigo.bunka.go.jp/guide.pdf (accessed 31 August 2016).

Burdelski, Matthew. 2010. Socializing politeness routines: Action, other-orientation, and embodiment in a Japanese preschool. *Journal of Pragmatics* 42(6). 1606–1621.

Burke, Deborah M. & Meredith A. Shafto. 2008. Language and aging. In F.I.M. Craik & T.A. Salthouse (eds.), *The handbook of aging and cognition* (Third edition), 373–443. New York: Psychology Press.

Button, Graham. 1987. Moving out of closings. In G. Button & J.R.E. Lee (eds.), *Talk and social organization*, 101–151. Clevedon: Multilingual Matters.

Cameron, Deborah. 1997. Performing gender identity: Young men's talk and the construction of heterosexual masculinity. In S. Johnson & U.H. Meinhof (eds.), *Language and masculinity*, 47–64. Oxford: Blackwell.

Campbell, John C. 2000. Changing meanings of frail old people and the Japanese welfare state. In S.O. Long (ed.), *Caring for the elderly in Japan and the US*, 82–97. London & New York: Routledge.

Candlin, Sally & Peter Roger (eds.). 2013. *Communication and professional relationships in healthcare practice*. Sheffield: Equinox.

Caporael, Linnda R. 1981. The paralanguage of care giving: Baby talk to the institutionalized aged. *Journal of Personality and Social Psychology* 40(5). 876–884.

Caporael, Linnda R., Marlene P. Lukaszewski & Glen H. Culbertson. 1983. Secondary baby talk: Judgements by institutionalized elderly and their caregivers. *Journal of Personality and Social Psychology* 44(4). 746–754.

Caris-Verhallen, Wilma M.C.M., Ingrid M. de Gruijter, Ada Kerkstra & Jozien M. Bensing. 1999. Factors related to nurse communication with elderly people. *Journal of Advanced Nursing* 30(5). 1106–1117.

Carpiac-Claver, Maria L. & Lené Levy-Storms. 2007. In a manner of speaking: Communication between nurse aides and older adults in long-term care settings. *Health Communication* 22(1). 59–67.

Chan, Engle A., Aled Jones, Sylvia Fung & Sui Chu Wu. 2011. Nurses' perception of time availability in patient communication in Hong Kong. *Journal of Clinical Nursing* 21(7/8). 1168–1177.

Clancy, Patricia M. 1986. The acquisition of communicative style in Japanese. In B.B. Schieffelin & E. Ochs (eds.), *Language socialization across cultures*, 213–250. Cambridge: Cambridge University Press.

Clark, Scott. 1992. The Japanese bath: Extraordinarily ordinary. In J.J. Tobin (ed.), *Re-made in Japan: Everyday life and consumer taste in a changing society*, 89–105. New Haven: Yale University Press.

Clyne, Michael, Catrin Norrby & Jane Warren. 2009. *Language and human relations: Styles of address in contemporary language*. Cambridge: Cambridge University Press.

Coates, Jennifer. 2004. *Women, men, and language: A sociolinguistic account of gender differences in language*. Harlow & New York: Pearson Longman.

Cook, Haruko M. 1997. The role of the Japanese *masu* form in caregiver–child conversation. *Journal of Pragmatics* 28(6). 695–718.

Cook, Haruko M. 1999. Situational meanings of Japanese social deixis: The mixed use of the *masu* and plain forms. *Journal of Linguistic Anthropology* 8(1). 87–110.

Cook, Haruko M. 2008. Style shifts in academic consultations. In K. Jones & T. Ono (eds.), *Style shifting in Japanese*, 9–38. Amsterdam & Philadelphia: Benjamins.

Coulmas, Florian. 2007. *Population decline and ageing in Japan: The social consequences*. London & New York: Routledge.

Coulmas, Florian, Harald Conrad, Annette Schad-Seifert & Gabriele Vogt (eds.). 2008. *The demographic challenge: A handbook about Japan*. Leiden & Boston: Brill.

Coupland, Justine. 2000. Introduction: Sociolinguistic perspectives on small talk. In J. Coupland (ed.), *Small talk*, 1–25. Essex: Pearson Education.

Coupland, Justine. 2009. Discourse, identity and change in mid-to-late life: Interdisciplinary perspectives on language and ageing. *Ageing & Society* 29. 849–861.

Coupland, Justine, Nikolas Coupland & Jeffrey D. Robinson. 1992. 'How are you?' Negotiating phatic communion. *Language in Society* 21(2). 207–230.

Coupland, Nikolas & Adam Jaworski (eds.). 1997. *Sociolinguistics: A reader and coursebook*. Basingstoke: Palgrave Macmillan.

Coupland, Nikolas & Virpi Ylänne-McEwen. 1993. Introduction: Discourse, institutions and the elderly. *Journal of Aging Studies* 7(3). 229–235.

Coupland, Nikolas & Virpi Ylänne-McEwen. 2000. Talk about the weather: Small talk, leisure talk and the travel industry. In J. Coupland (ed.), *Small talk*, 163–182. Essex: Pearson Education.

Coupland, Nikolas & Virpi Ylänne-McEwen. 2006. The sociolinguistics of ageing. In U. Ammon, N. Dittmar, K.J. Mattheier & P. Trudgill (eds.), *Sociolinguistics: An international handbook of the science of language and society* (Vol.3), 2334–2340. Berlin & New York: De Gruyter.

Craven, Alexandra & Jonathan Potter. 2010. Directives: Contingency and entitlement in action. *Discourse Studies* 12(4). 419–442.

Cross, Simon & Barbara Bagilhole. 2002. Girls' jobs for the boys? Men, masculinity and non-traditional occupations. *Gender, Work and Organization* 9(2). 204–226.

Culpeper, Jonathan. 2011. *Impoliteness: Using language to cause offence*. Cambridge: Cambridge University Press.

Curl, Traci S. & Paul Drew. 2008. Contingency and action: A comparison of two forms of requesting. *Research on Language and Social Interaction* 41(2). 129–153.

Dalton-Puffer, Christiane. 2005. Negotiating interpersonal meanings in naturalistic classroom discourse: Directives in content-and-language-integrated classrooms. *Journal of Pragmatics* 37(8). 1275–1293.

Daniel, Michael & Andrew Spencer. 2009. The vocative – An outlier case. In A. Malchukov & A. Spencer (eds.), *The Oxford handbook of case*, 626–634. Oxford: Oxford University Press.

David, Oana. 2009. *Teineigo* and style mixing: Formality variation in the interview register and application of conversation analysis theory. Master's thesis, University of Oxford. http://linguistics.berkeley.edu/~oana/teineigo.pdf (accessed 31 August 2016).

Davidson, Judy. 1984. Subsequent versions of invitations, offers, requests, and proposals dealing with potential or actual rejection. In J.M. Atkinson & J. Heritage (eds.), *Structures of social action*, 102–128. Cambridge: Cambridge University Press.

Davis, Boyd, Margaret Maclagan & Dena Shenk. 2016. The silent violence of marginalization and teasing in dementia care residences. *Journal of Language Aggression and Conflict* 4(1). 35–61.

Davis, Boyd & Charlene Pope. 2010. Institutionalized ghosting: Policy contexts and language use in the process of erasing the person with Alzheimer's. *Language Policy* 9(1). 29–44.

Dickey, Eleanor. 1997. Forms of address and terms of reference. *Journal of Linguistics* 33(2). 225–274.

Dijkstra, Katinka, Michelle Bourgeois, Lou Burgio & Rebecca Allen. 2002. Effects of a communication intervention on the discourse of nursing home residents with dementia and their nursing assistants. *Journal of Medical Speech–Language Pathology* 10(2). 43–58.

Drew, Paul & John Heritage. 1992. Analyzing talk at work: An introduction. In P. Drew & J. Heritage (eds.), *Talk at work: Interaction in institutional settings*, 1–65. Cambridge: Cambridge University Press.

Duffy, Mignon, Clare L. Stacey & Amy Armenia. 2015. Epilogue. In M. Duffy, A. Armenia & C.L. Stacey (eds.), *Caring on the clock: The complexities and contradictions of paid care work*, 287–291. New Brunswick: Rutgers University Press.

Edwards, Helen, Deanne Gaskill, Fran Sanders, Elizabeth Forster, Paul Morrison, Rosanne Fleming, Sandra McClure & Helen Chapman. 2003. Resident–staff interactions: A challenge for quality residential aged care. *Australasian Journal on Ageing* 22(1). 31–37.

Ehlich, Konrad & Jochen Rehbein. 1980. Sprache in Institutionen. In H.P. Althaus, H. Henne & H.E. Wieland (eds.), *Lexikon der Germanistischen Linguistik* (Second edition), 338–345. Tübingen: Niemeyer.

Ellis, Rod. 1992. Learning to communicate in the classroom: A study of two language learners' requests. *Studies in Second Language Acquisition* 14(1). 1–23.

Endō, Orie & Reiko Saegusa. 2015. *Yasashiku iikaeyō kaigo no kotoba* [Let's use more easily understandable care language]. Tokyo: Sanseidō.

Endo, Tomoko & Akira Takada. 2016. Iu koto kikinasai: kōi shiji ni okeru taiō no tsuikyū to sekinin no keisei [Listen to what I say: Pursuing reactions to action commands and the formation of responsibility]. In A. Takada, Y. Shimada & R. Kawashima (eds.), *Kosodate no kaiwa bunseki: sekinin wa dō sodatsu ka* [Conversation analysis of childrearing: How responsibility is brought up], 55–75. Kyoto: Showado.

Engbersen, Agnes M. 2009. Communication in a Dutch caring institution. Paper presented at the conference 'Communication in Institutional Elderly Care: Cross-cultural Perspectives'. German Institute for Japanese Studies, Tokyo, 1–2 October.

Engbersen, Agnes. M. 2013. The use of the Dutch particle *NOU* in care services with elderly. Unpublished manuscript.

Enyo, Yumiko. 2015. Contexts and meanings of Japanese speech styles: A case of hierarchical identity construction among Japanese college students. *Pragmatics* 25(3). 345–367.

Erickson, Rebecca J. & Clare L. Stacey. 2013. Attending to mind and body: Engaging the complexity of emotion practice among caring professionals. In A.A. Grandey, J.M. Diefendorff & D.E. Rupp (eds.), *Emotional labor in the 21st century: Diverse perspectives on the psychology of emotion regulation at work*, 175–196. New York: Routledge.

Ervin-Tripp, Susan. 1972. On sociolinguistic rules: Alternation and co-occurrence. In J.J. Gumperz & D.H. Hymes (eds.), *Directions in sociolinguistics: The ethnography of communication*, 213–250. New York: Holt, Rinehart & Winston.

Ervin-Tripp, Susan. 1976. 'Is Sybil there?' The structure of some American English directives. *Language in Society* 5(1). 25–66.

Ervin-Tripp, Susan, Jiansheng Guo & Martin Lampert. 1990. Politeness and persuasion in children's control acts. *Journal of Pragmatics* 14(2). 307–331.

Fairhurst, Eileen. 1978. Talk and the elderly in institutions. Paper presented to the annual conference of the British Society of Social and Behavioural Gerontology, Edinburgh, 14–16 September.

Fairhurst, Eileen. 1981. A sociological study of the rehabilitation of the elderly in an urban hospital. Doctoral dissertation, University of Leeds.

Félix-Brasdefer, J. César. 2015. *The language of service encounters: A pragmatic-discursive approach*. Cambridge: Cambridge University Press.

Fiehler, Reinhard. 1980. Kommunikation und ihre Rolle in verschiedenen Typen von Tätigkeitszusammenhängen. In G. Tschauder & E. Weigand (eds.), *Perspektive: textextern*, 63–72. Tübingen: Niemeyer. http://ids-pub.bsz-bw.de/frontdoor/index/index/docId/717 (accessed 31 August 2016).

Finlay, W. Mick L., Charles Antaki & Chris Walton. 2008. Saying no to the staff: An analysis of refusals in a home for people with severe communication difficulties. *Sociology of Health and Illness* 30(1). 55–75.

Flöck, Ilka. 2016. *Requests in American and British English: A contrastive multi-method analysis*. Amsterdam & Philadelphia: Benjamins.

Formentelli, Maicol. 2009. Address strategies in a British academic setting. *Pragmatics* 19(2). 179–196.

Fukada, Kōichirō. 2009. Kaigo to iu komyunikēshon: kankei no hitaishōsei o megutte [Care communication: Focusing on relational asymmetries]. *Fukushi shakaigaku kenkyū* 6. 82–101.

Fukuda, Chie. 2005. Children's use of the *masu* form in play scenes. *Journal of Pragmatics* 37(7). 1037–1058.

Fukushima, Saeko. 2003. *Requests and culture: Politeness in British English and Japanese*. Bern & New York: Lang.

Fukushima, Saeko. 2009. Request strategies among equals in Japanese. *Tsuru University Graduate School Review* 13. 13–32. http://ci.nii.ac.jp/naid/110007129832 (accessed 31 August 2016).

Furukawa, Hidetoshi, Kazuko Kunitake & Fusako Noguchi. 2002. Gurūp hōmu ni okeru chihōsei rōjin no kōdō bunseki [Behaviour analysis of group home residents with dementia]. *Kenritsu Nagasaki Shīboruto daigaku kango eiyō gakubu kiyō* 2. 73–83. http://ci.nii.ac.jp/naid/110000039580/ (accessed 31 August 2016).

Furuta, Tomoko & Kaoru Horie. 2011. Kaigo genba ni okeru nyūyoku bamen de no kaijosha to riyōsha to no kankei kōchiku: supīchi reberu shifuto to pojitibu poraitonesu sutoratejī kara no kōsatsu [Relationship building between care worker and resident in care settings during bathing: Examining speech level shift and positive politeness strategies]. *Nihon goyōron gakkai taikai happyō ronbunshū* 7. 245–248.

Furuta, Tomoko & Kaoru Horie. 2014. Nyūyoku kaijo bamen ni okeru supīchi reberu to supīchi reberu shifuto: sono jittai to kinō [Speech level and speech level shift during bathing support: State and functions]. Unpublished manuscript.

Garcia, Angela Cora. 2013. *An introduction to interaction: Understanding talk in formal and informal settings.* London & New York: Bloomsbury.

Garvey, Catherine. 1975. Requests and responses in children's speech. *Journal of Child Language* 2(1). 41–63.

Geyer, Naomi. 2008a. *Discourse and politeness: Ambivalent face in Japanese.* London & New York: Continuum.

Geyer, Naomi. 2008b. Interpersonal functions of style shift: The use of plain and *masu* forms in faculty meetings. In K. Jones & T. Ono (eds.), *Style shifting in Japanese*, 39–70. Amsterdam & Philadelphia: Benjamins.

Gibb, Heather. 1990. *'This is what we have to do – Are you okay?' Nurses' speech with elderly nursing home residents* (Research Monograph Series 1). Geelong: Deakin University.

Gibb, Heather & Bart O'Brien. 1990. Jokes and reassurance are not enough: Ways in which nurses relate through conversation with elderly clients. *Journal of Advanced Nursing* 15(12). 1389–1401.

Gibbon, Dafydd. 1981. Idiomaticity and functional variation: A case study of international amateur radio talk. *Language in Society* 8(1). 21–42.

Giles, Howard (ed.). 2016. *Communication accommodation theory: Negotiating personal relationships and social identities across contexts.* Cambridge: Cambridge University Press.

Giles, Howard, Justine Coupland & Nikolas Coupland. 1991. *Contexts of accommodation: Developments in applied sociolinguistics.* Cambridge: Cambridge University Press.

Glenn, Phillip. 2003. *Laughter in interaction.* Cambridge: Cambridge University Press.

Goffman, Erving. 1961. *Asylums: Essays on the social situation of mental patients and other inmates.* New York: Random House.

Goffman, Erving. 1967. *Interaction ritual: Essays on face-to-face behavior.* New York: Doubleday.

Goffman, Erving. 1981. *Forms of talk.* Oxford: Blackwell.

Golato, Andrea & Zsuzsanna Fagyal. 2008. Comparing single and double sayings of the German response token *ja* and the role of prosody: A conversation analytical perspective. *Research on Language and Social Interaction* 41(3). 241–270.

Goldberg, Julia A. 1990. Interrupting the discourse on interruptions: An analysis in terms of relationally neutral, power- and rapport-oriented acts. *Journal of Pragmatics* 14(6). 883–903.

Goodwin, Charles. 1984. Notes on story structure and the organization of participation. In J.M. Atkinson & J. Heritage (eds.), *Structures of social action*, 225–246. Cambridge: Cambridge University Press.

Goodwin, Marjorie H. 1980. Directive–response speech sequences in girls' and boys' task activities. In S. McConnell-Ginet, R. Borker & N. Furman (eds.), *Women and language in literature and society*, 157–173. New York: Praeger.

Goodwin, Marjorie H. 1988. Cooperation and competition across girls' play activities. In A.D. Todd & S. Fisher (eds.), *Gender and discourse: The power of talk*, 55–94. Norwood: Ablex.

Goodwin, Marjorie H. & Asta Cekaite. 2013. Calibration in directive/response sequences in family interaction. *Journal of Pragmatics* 46(1). 122–138.

Goto, Noriko, Satoshi Kumasaka, Noriko Sanpei, Eunhee Sawa, Miho Saitō & Ryūko Yamakami. 2010. Kaigo hoken shisetsu riyōsha to ryūgakusei no kaiwa no bunseki: Yamagata chiikigo no rikai o chūshin ni [Analysing talk between care facility users and foreign students: Focus on understanding the Yamagata dialect] *Yamagata tanki daigaku kiyō* 42. 13–26. http://id.nii.ac.jp/1369/00000022/ (accessed 31 August 2016).

Goto, Shihoko. 2014. Tackling Japan's demographic time bomb. *Georgetown Journal of International Affairs*, 22 August. http://journal.georgetown.edu/tackling-japans-demographic-time-bomb/ (accessed 31 August 2016).

Grainger, Karen. 1990. Care and control: Interactional management in nursing the elderly. In R. Clark, N. Fairclough, R. Ivanic, N. McLeod, J. Thomas & P. Meara (eds.), *Language and power*, 147–157. London: Centre for Information and Language Teaching.

Grainger, Karen. 1993a. The discourse of elderly care. Dissertation thesis, University of Wales.

Grainger, Karen. 1993b. 'That's a lovely bath, dear': Reality construction in the discourse of elderly care. *Journal of Aging Studies* 7(3). 247–262.

Grainger, Karen. 1998. Reality orientation in institutions for the elderly: The perspective from interactional sociolinguistics. *Journal of Aging Studies* 12(1). 39–56.

Grainger, Karen. 2004a. Verbal play on the hospital ward: Solidarity or power? *Multilingua* 23(1/2). 39–59.

Grainger, Karen. 2004b. Communication and the institutionalized elderly. In J.F. Nussbaum & J. Coupland (eds.), *Handbook of communication and aging research* (Second edition), 479–497. Mahwah & London: Erlbaum.

Grainger, Karen, Karen Atkinson & Nikolas Coupland. 1990. *Responding to the elderly: Troubles talk in the caring context.* In H. Giles, N. Coupland & J. Wiemann (eds.), *Communication, health and the elderly*, 192–212. Manchester: Manchester University Press.

Gubrium, Jaber. 1975. *Living and dying at Murray Manor.* New York: St. Martin's Press.

Haddington, Pentti, Tiina Keisanen, Lorenza Mondada & Maurice Nevile (eds.). 2014a. *Multiactivity in social interaction: Beyond multitasking.* Amsterdam & Philadelphia: Benjamins.

Haddington, Pentti, Tiina Keisanen, Lorenza Mondada & Maurice Nevile. 2014b. Introduction. In P. Haddington, T. Keisanen, L. Mondada & M. Nevile (eds.), *Multiactivity in social interaction: Beyond multitasking*, 3–32. Amsterdam & Philadelphia: Benjamins.

Hallberg, Ingalill R., Astrid Norberg & Kristina Johnsson. 1993. Verbal interaction during the lunch-meal between caregivers and vocally disruptive demented patients. *American Journal of Alzheimer's Care and Related Disorders & Research* 8(3). 26–32.

Hamilton, Heidi E. 1994. *Conversations with an Alzheimer's patient.* Cambridge: Cambridge University Press.

Hamilton, Heidi E. & Toshiko Hamaguchi. 2015. Discourse and aging. In D. Tannen, H.E. Hamilton & D. Schiffrin (eds.), *Handbook of discourse analysis*, 705–727. Malden: Wiley-Blackwell.

Harada, Sayo. 2014. Effects and issues in a coping skill training program for certified caregivers. *Nihon kenkō igaku gakkaishi* 22(4). 253–263. http://ci.nii.ac.jp/naid/110009688333/ (accessed 31 August 2016).

Harris, Sandra. 2003. Politeness and power: Making and responding to requests in institutional settings. *Text* 23(1). 27–52.

Hartmann, Dietrich. 1972. Der Gebrauch von Namen und Personenbezeichnungen als Ausdruck sozialer Beziehungen in einer Kleingruppe. In K. Hyldgaard-Jensen (ed.), *Linguistik: Referate des 6. linguistischen Kolloquiums*, 285–306. Frankfurt: Athenaeum.

Hasegawa, Yoko. 2010. *Soliloquy in Japanese and English*. Amsterdam & Philadelphia: Benjamins.

Hasegawa, Yoko. 2015. *Japanese: A linguistic introduction*. Cambridge: Cambridge University Press.

Haugh, Michael. 2007. The discursive challenge to politeness research: An interactional perspective. *Journal of Politeness Research* 3. 295–317.

Heath, Christian. 1986. *Body movement and speech in medical interaction*. Cambridge: Cambridge University Press.

Heikes, E. Joel. 1991. When men are in the minority: The case of men in nursing. *The Sociological Quarterly* 32(3). 389–401.

Heinemann, Trine. 2006. Will you or can't you? Displaying entitlement in interrogative requests. *Journal of Pragmatics* 38(7). 1081–1104.

Heinemann, Trine. 2007. Professional self-disclosure: When the home help talks about herself. In C. Kerbrat-Orecchioni & V. Traverso (eds.), *Confidence/dévoilement de soi dans l'interaction*, 325–342. Tübingen: Niemeyer.

Heinemann, Trine. 2008. Participation and exclusion in third party complaints. *Journal of Pragmatics* 41(12). 2435–2451.

Heinemann, Trine. 2009a. Managing unavoidable conflicts in caretaking of the elderly: Humor as a mitigating resource. *International Journal of the Sociology of Language* 200. 103–127.

Heinemann, Trine. 2009b. Two answers to inapposite inquiries. In J. Sidnell (ed.), *Conversation analysis: Comparative perspectives*, 159–186. Cambridge: Cambridge University Press.

Heinemann, Trine. 2011. From home to institution: Roles, relations and the loss of autonomy in caretaking of the elderly in Denmark. In P. Backhaus (ed.), *Communication in elderly care: Cross-cultural perspectives*, 90–111. London & New York: Continuum.

Heinrich, Patrick. 2015. The study of politeness and women's language in Japan. In D. Smakman & P. Heinrich (eds.), *Globalising sociolinguistics: Challenging and expanding theory*, 178–193. London & New York: Routledge.

Henzl, Vera M. 1989. Linguistic means of social distancing in physician–patient interaction. In W. von Raffler-Engel (ed.), *Doctor–patient interaction*, 77–91. Amsterdam & Philadelphia: Benjamins.

Heritage, John. 1984a. *Garfinkel and ethnomethodology*. Cambridge: Polity Press.

Heritage, John. 1984b. A change-of-state token and aspects of its sequential placement. In J.M. Atkinson & J. Heritage (eds.), *Structures of social action*, 299–345. Cambridge: Cambridge University Press.

Heritage, John. 1997. Conversation analysis and institutional talk: Analysing data. In D. Silverman (ed.), *Qualitative research: Theory, method and practice*, 160–182. London & Thousand Oaks: Sage.

Heritage, John. 2004. Conversation analysis and institutional talk. In R. Sanders & K. Fitch (eds.), *Handbook of language and social interaction*, 103–146. Mahwah: Erlbaum.

Heritage, John & Steve Clayman. 2010. *Talk in action: Interactions, identities, and institutions.* Chichester & Malden: Wiley-Blackwell.

Heritage, John & Jeffrey D. Robinson. 2006. Accounting for the visit: Giving reasons for seeking medical care. In J. Heritage & D.W. Maynard (eds.), *Communication in medical care: Interaction between primary care physicians and patients,* 48–85. Cambridge & New York: Cambridge University Press.

Herzberger, Patricia. 1999. 'Dem kannst zuereden wiest willst, er tut nix': Handlungsaufforderungen in der Altenpflege. *Wiener Linguistische Gazette* 66. 32–53. https://www.univie.ac.at/linguistics/publications/wlg/661999/WLG661999Herzberger.pdf (accessed 31 August 2016).

Hewison, Alistair. 1995. Nurses' power in interactions with patients. *Journal of Advanced Nursing* 21(1). 75–82.

Hinata, Shigeo. 1980. Danwa ni okeru 'hai' to 'ee' no kinō [*Hai* and *ee* in discourse]. *Kokuritsu kokugo kenkyūjo kenkyū hōkoku* 65(2). 215–229.

Hochschild, Arlie Russel. 1983. *The managed heart: Commercialization of human feeling* (Twentieth anniversary edition with a new afterword, 2003). Berkeley: University of California Press.

Holmes, Janet. 1983. The structure of teacher's directives. In J.C. Richards & R.W. Schmidt (eds.), *Language and communication,* 89–115. London: Longman.

Holmes, Janet. 1995. *Women, men and politeness.* London: Longman.

Holmes, Janet. 2000. Doing collegiality and keeping control at work: Small talk in government departments. In J. Coupland (ed.), *Small talk,* 32–61. Essex: Pearson Education.

Holmes, Janet. 2012. Politeness in intercultural discourse and communication. In C.B. Paulston, S.F. Kiesling & E.S. Rangel (eds.), *The handbook of intercultural discourse and communication,* 205–228. Malden: Blackwell.

Hook, Donald D. 1984. First names and titles as solidarity and power semantics in English. *International Review of Applied Linguistics* 22(3). 183–189.

Horii, Mitsutoshi. 2014. Why do the Japanese wear masks? A short historical review. *Electronic Journal of Contemporary Japanese Studies* 14(2). http://www.japanesestudies.org.uk/ejcjs/vol14/iss2/horii.html (accessed 31 August 2016).

Hosoma, Hiromichi. 2016. *Kaigo suru karada* [Bodies doing care]. Tokyo: Igaku shoin.

Hudson, Mutsuko Endo. 2011. Student honorifics usage in conversations with professors. *Journal of Pragmatics* 43(15). 3689–3706.

Hummert, Mary Lee & Debra C. Mazloff. 2001. Older adults' response to patronizing advice: Balancing politeness and identity in context. *Journal of Language and Social Psychology* 20(1/2). 168–196.

Hummert, Mary Lee & Ellen Bouchard Ryan. 1996. Toward understanding variations in patronizing talk addressed to older adults: Psycholinguistic features of care and control. *International Journal of Psycholinguistics* 12. 149–169.

Hutchby, Ian & Robin Wooffitt. 2008. *Conversation analysis: Principles, practices and applications* (Second edition). Oxford: Polity Press.

Ide, Sachiko. 1982. Japanese sociolinguistics: Politeness and women's language. *Lingua* 57(2). 357–385.

Ide, Sachiko. 1989. Formal forms and discernment: Two neglected aspects of universals of linguistic politeness. *Multilingua* 8(2/3). 223–248.

Ide, Sachiko & Megumi Yoshida. 1999. Sociolinguistics: Honorifics and gender differences. In N. Tsujimura (ed.), *The handbook of Japanese linguistics,* 444–480. Malden & Oxford: Blackwell.

Ikuta, Shoko. 1983. Speech level shift and conversational strategy in Japanese discourse. *Language Sciences* 5(1). 37–53.

Ilie, Cornelia. 2010. Strategic uses of parliamentary forms of address: The case of the U.K. Parliament and the Swedish Riksdag. *Journal of Pragmatics* 42(4). 885–911.

Inoue, Miyako. 2006. *Vicarious language: Gender and linguistic modernity in Japan.* Berkeley: University of California Press.

IPSS (National Institute of Population and Social Security Research). 2014. Social security in Japan. http://www.ipss.go.jp/s-info/e/ssj2014/pdf/SSJ2014.pdf (accessed 31 August 2016).

IPSS (National Institute of Population and Social Security Research). 2016. Jinkō tōkei shiryōshū 2016 [Reference material on population statistics]. http://www.ipss.go.jp/syoushika/tohkei/Popular/Popular2016.asp?chap=2 (accessed 31 August 2016).

Irish, Julie & Judith A. Hall. 1995. Interruptive patterns in medical visits: The effects of role, status and gender. *Social Science & Medicine* 41(6). 873–881.

Ishikawa, Minako. 1991. Iconicity in discourse: The case of repetition. *Text* 11(4). 553–580.

Ishizaki, Akiko. 2000. Denwa renraku no kaiwa ni okeru supīchi reberu shifuto [Speech level shifts in telephone conversation]. *Gengo bunka to Nihongo kyōiku* 19. 62–74. http://ci.nii.ac.jp/naid/120002836183 (accessed 31 August 2016).

Isosävi, Johanna & Hanna Lappalainen. 2015. First names in Starbucks: A clash of cultures? In C. Norrby & C. Wide (eds.), *Address practice as social action: European perspectives*, 97–118. Houndmills: Palgrave Macmillan.

Israeli, Alina. 1997. Syntactic reduplication in Russian: A cooperative principle device in dialogues. *Journal of Pragmatics* 27(5). 587–609.

Itakura, Hiroko. 2015. Constructing Japanese men's multidimensional identities: A case study of mixed-gender talk. *Pragmatics* 25(2). 179–203.

Iwasaki, Shoichi. 2013. *Japanese* (Revised edition). Amsterdam & Philadelphia: Benjamins.

Jacquemet, Marco. 1994. T-offenses and metapragmatic attacks: Strategies of interaction dominance. *Discourse & Society* 5(3). 297–319.

Jakobson, Roman. 1971. Zur Struktur des russischen Verbums. In R. Jakobson, *Word and language*, 3–15. The Hague & Paris: Mouton.

Janes, Angela. 2000. The interaction of style-shift and particle use in Japanese dialogue. *Journal of Pragmatics* 32(12). 1823–1853.

Jansson, Gunilla. 2016. You're doing everything just fine: Praise in residential care settings. *Discourse Studies* 18(1). 64–86.

Jansson, Gunilla & Charlotta Plejert. 2014. Taking a shower: Managing a potentially imposing activity in dementia care. *Journal of Interactional Research in Communication Disorders* 5(1). 27–62.

Jaworski, Adam & Dariusz Galasiński. 2000. Vocative address forms and ideological legitimization in political debates. *Discourse Studies* 2(1). 35–53.

Jefferson, Gail. 1984a. Notes on some orderlinesses of overlap onset. In V. D'Urso & P. Leonardi (eds.), *Discourse analysis and natural rhetoric*, 11–38. Padua: Cleup Editore.

Jefferson, Gail. 1984b. Notes on a systematic deployment of the acknowledgment tokens 'yeah' and 'mm hm'. *Papers in Linguistics* 17(2). 197–216.

Jefferson, Gail. 1989. Preliminary notes on a possible metric which provides for a 'standard maximum' silence of approximately one second in conversation. In D. Roger &

P. Bull (eds.), *Conversation: An interdisciplinary perspective*, 166–196. Clevedon: Multilingual Matters.

Jefferson, Gail. 2004. Glossary of transcript symbols with an introduction. In G.H. Lerner (ed.), *Conversation analysis: Studies from the first generation*, 13–23. Amsterdam & Philadelphia: Benjamins.

Jenike, Brenda Robb. 2003. Parent care and shifting family obligations in urban Japan. In J. Traphagan & J. Knight (eds.), *Demographic change and the family in Japan's aging society*, 177–201. Albany: State University of New York Press.

JFKC (Japan Foundation Japanese-Language Institute, Kansai). 2009. *Gaikokujin no tame no kango/kaigo yōgoshū* [Nursing and care glossary for foreigners]. Tokyo: Bonjinsha.

Jones, Daniel C. & Gemma M.M. van Amelsvoort Jones. 1986. Communication patterns between nursing staff and the ethnic elderly in a long-term care facility. *Journal of Advanced Nursing* 11(3). 265–272.

Jones, Kimberly. 1992. A question of context: Directive use at a Morris team meeting. *Language in Society* 21(3). 427–445.

Jones, Kimberly & Tsuyoshi Ono. 2008. The messy reality of style shifting. In K. Jones & T. Ono (eds.), *Style shifting in Japanese*, 1–7. Amsterdam & Philadelphia: Benjamins.

Kambe, Satoshi. 2015. Kaigo rōjin fukushi shisetsu ni okeru wakate kaigo shokuin no ninchishō kōreisha to no komyunikēshon ni tai suru ninshiki [Young care workers' awareness of communication with dementia patients in a care facility]. *Ōsaka Ōtani daigaku kiyō* 49. 1–9.

Kaneda, Chikako. 2005. Shintaiteki jiritsudo no takai chihōsei kōreisha no kōdō bunseki ni kan suru kenkyū: jūraigata tokubetsu yōgo rōjin hōmu ni okeru taimu sutadi o tōshite [Research on action analysis of dementia patients with a high degree of independence: A time study in an old-type nursing home]. *Iryō fukushi kenkyū* 1. 57–65. http://ci.nii.ac.jp/naid/110006219878 (accessed 31 August 2016).

Kasper, Gabriele (ed.). 2006. *Multilingua* 25(3). Special issue on Politeness in Interaction.

Kayser-Jones, Jeanie S. 1981. *Old, alone and neglected: Care of the aged in Scotland and the United States*. Berkeley: University of California Press.

Keevallik, Leelo. 2010. Social action of syntactic reduplication. *Journal of Pragmatics* 42(3). 800–824.

Keisanen, Tiina, Mirka Rauniomaa & Pentti Haddington. 2014. Suspending action: From simultaneous to consecutive ordering of multiple courses of action. In P. Haddington, T. Keisanen, L. Mondada & M. Nevile (eds.), *Multiactivity in social interaction: Beyond multitasking*, 109–133. Amsterdam & Philadelphia: Benjamins.

Kim, Sung-Ill, Kazuki Nakajima, Kanako Nakamura, Yuji Higashi, Masayuki Nambu, Toshiro Fujimoto & Toshiyo Tamura. 2000. Kōreisha no hatsuwa o unagasu kaiwa shisutemu [Interactive system for encouraging older people's utterances]. *Denshi jōhō tsūshin gakkai gijutsu kenkyū hōkoku* 100(521). 85–90.

Kingston, Jeff. 2011. *Japan in transformation, 1945–2010* (Second edition). Harlow: Longman.

Kinoshita, Yasuhito & Christie W. Kiefer. 1992. *Refuge of the honored: Social organization in a Japanese retirement community*. Berkeley: University of California Press.

Kinsui, Satoshi. 2003. *Vācharu Nihongo: yakuwarigo no nazo* [Virtual Japanese: The riddle of role language]. Tokyo: Iwanami.

Kinsui, Satoshi (ed.). 2007. *Yakuwarigo kenkyū no chihei* [Horizons of role language research]. Tokyo: Kuroshio.

Kitagawa, Chisato. 1980. Saying 'yes' in Japanese. *Journal of Pragmatics* 4(2). 105–120.

Kitamoto, Keiko. 2006. Sōsharu wāku ni okeru komyunikēshon bunseki: tokubetsu yōgo rōjin hōmu ni okeru seikatsu bamen o chūshin ni [Analysis of communication in social work: Everyday situations in a nursing home]. *Jōsai kokusai daigaku daigakuin kiyō* 9. 49–64.

Kitamoto, Keiko. 2007. Sōsharu wāku ni kan suru kenkyū: seikatsu shisetsu ni okeru sōsharu wāku ni shōten o atete [Research on social work: Focus on social work in a community facility]. Doctoral dissertation, Taisho University, Tokyo.

Kitayama, Tamaki. 2013. The distribution and characteristics of Japanese vocatives in business situations. *Pragmatics* 23(3). 447–479.

Kitwood, Tom. 1997. *Dementia reconsidered: The person comes first.* Berkshire: Open University Press.

Kobayashi, Shusuke. 2001. Japanese mother–child relationships: Skill acquisition during the preschool years. In H. Shimizu & R. Levine (eds.), *Japanese frames of mind: Cultural perspectives on human development*, 111–142. New York: Cambridge University Press.

Koester, Almut J. 2004. Relational sequences in workplace genres. *Journal of Pragmatics* 36(8). 1405–1428.

Koike, Taeko. 2000. Zaitaku ni okeru chihōsei kōreisha ni tai suru kaigosha no taido to komyunikēshon no jittai [Attitudes and communication problems faced by care workers towards homebound elderly with dementia]. *Ōtsuma joshi daigaku ningen kankei gakubu kiyō* 1. 193–206.

Komatsu, Mitsuyo. 2005. Kaigo rōjin fukushi shisetsu ni okeru ninchishō kōreisha e no kea gijutsu ni kan suru kaigo sutaffu no jūyōsei ninshiki to jissen hindo no hikaku [Comparing staff's recognition of care techniques and their frequency of occurrence in a dementia care facility]. *Hyōron shakai kagaku* 77. 99–113. http://ci.nii.ac.jp/naid/110007391077 (accessed 31 August 2016).

Komatsu, Mitsuyo, Yasuhiro Kuroki & Yasuko Okayama. 2003. Kaigo rōjin fukushi shisetsu ni okeru chihōsei kōreisha kea gijutsu no meikakuka: kaigo sutaffu no nichijō seikatsu enjo bamen e no sanka kansatsu ni yoru shitsuteki bunseki [Clarification of techniques in institutional dementia care: Qualitative analysis of everyday life care based on participant observation]. *Nihon chihō kea gakkaishi* 2(1). 56–67.

Korkiakangas, Terhi, Sharon-Marie Weldon, Jeff Bezemer & Roger Kneebone. 2016. 'Coming up!' Why verbal acknowledgement matters in the operating theatre. In S.J. White & J.A. Cartmill (eds.), *Communication in surgical practice*, 234–256. Sheffield: Equinox.

Kuiper, Koenraad & Marie Flindall. 2000. Social rituals, formulaic speech and small talk at the supermarket checkout. In J. Coupland (ed.), *Small talk*, 183–207. Essex: Pearson Education.

Kuramochi, Masuko. 2009. Shin-keigo 'su' no shiyō bamen no kakudai to kinō no henka [Spread of usage and functional change of the novel honorific *su*]. *Meikai Nihongo* 14. 25–35.

Kuroshima, Satomi. 2010. Another look at the service encounter: Progressivity, intersubjectivity, and trust in a Japanese sushi restaurant. *Journal of Pragmatics* 42(3). 856–869.

Lakoff, Robin. 1975. *Language and woman's place.* New York: Harper & Row.

Lanceley, Anne. 1985. Use of controlling language in the rehabilitation of the elderly. *Journal of Advanced Nursing* 10(2). 125–135.

Länsisalmi, Rikka. 2001. You and I in Japanese: What do 'personal pronouns' do in Japanese discourse? *SKY Journal of Linguistics* 14. 121–150.

Laver, John. 1975. Communicative functions of phatic communion. In A. Kendon, R.M. Harris & M.R. Key (eds.), *Organization of behavior in face-to-face interaction*, 215–238. The Hague: Mouton.

Leech, Geoffrey. 1999. The distribution and functions of vocatives. In H. Hasselgård & S. Oksefjell (eds.), *Out of corpora*, 107–118. Amsterdam: Rodopi.

Lerner, Gene H. 2004. Collaborative turn sequences. In G.H. Lerner (ed.), *Conversation analysis: Studies from the first generation*, 225–256. Amsterdam & Philadelphia: Benjamins.

Li, Han Z., Zhi Zhang, Young-Ok Yum, Juanita Lundgren & Jasrit S. Pahal. 2008. Interruption and patient satisfaction in resident–patient consultations. *Health Education* 108(5). 411–427.

Li, Li & Wen Ma. 2016. Request sequence in Chinese public service calls. *Discourse Studies* 18(3). 269–285.

Liddicoat, Anthony J. 2004. The projectability of turn constructional units and the role of prediction in listening. *Discourse Studies* 6(4). 449–469.

Liddicoat, Anthony J. 2007. *An introduction to conversation analysis.* London & New York: Continuum.

Lie, John. 2000. The discourse of Japaneseness. In M. Douglass & G.S. Roberts (eds.), *Japan and global migration: Foreign workers and the advent of a multicultural society*, 70–90. London & New York: Routledge.

Linde, Charlotte. 1988. The quantitative study of communicative success: Politeness and accidents in aviation discourse. *Language in Society* 17(3). 375–399.

Lindström, Anna. 2005. Language as social action: A study of how senior citizens request assistance with practical tasks in the Swedish home help service. In A. Hakulinen & M. Selting (eds.), *Syntax and lexis in conversation: Studies on the use of linguistic resources in talk-in-interaction*, 209–230. Amsterdam & Philadelphia: Benjamins.

Linhart, Sepp. 1997. Does *oyakōkō* still exist in present-day Japan? In S. Formanek & S. Linhart (eds.), *Aging: Asian concepts and experiences past and present*, 297–328. Vienna: Verlag der Österreichischen Wissenschaften.

Lipman, Alan, Robert Slater & Howard Harris. 1979. The quality of verbal interaction in homes for old people. *Gerontology* 25(5). 275–284.

Lubinski, Rosemary. 1988. A model for intervention: Communication skills, effectiveness, and opportunity. In B. Shadden (ed.), *Communication behavior and aging*, 294–308. Baltimore: Williams & Wilkins.

Lubinski, Rosemary. 1995. State-of-the-art perspectives on communication in nursing homes. *Topics in Language Disorders* 15(2). 1–19.

Lupton, Ben. 2000. Maintaining masculinity: Men who do women's work. *British Journal of Management* 11. 33–48.

Lyman, Karen A. 1988. Infantilization of elders: Day care for Alzheimer's Disease victims. In D.C. Wertz (ed.), *Research in the sociology of health care* (Vol.7), 71–104. Greenwich: JAI Press.

Macaulay, Ronald K.S. 2005. *Talk that counts: Age, gender, and social class differences in discourse.* Oxford & New York: Oxford University Press.

Maclagan, Margaret & Annabel Grant. 2011. Care of people with Alzheimer's Disease in New Zealand: Supporting the telling of life stories. In P. Backhaus (ed.),

Communication in eldercare: Cross-cultural perspectives, 62–89. London & New York: Continuum.

Macleod-Clark, Jill. 1982. Nurse–patient verbal interaction: An analysis of conversations in selected surgical wards. Doctoral dissertation, University of London.

Major, George & Janet Holmes. 2008. How do nurses describe health care procedures? Analysing nurse–patient interaction in a hospital ward. *Australian Journal of Advanced Nursing* 25(4). 58–70.

Makoni, Sinfree & Karen Grainger. 2002. Comparative gerontolinguistics: Characterizing discourses in caring institutions in South Africa and the United Kingdom. *Journal of Social Issues* 58(4). 805–824.

Malinowski, Bronislaw. 1923. The problem of meaning in primitive languages. In C.K. Ogden & I.A. Richards (eds.), *The meaning of meaning: A Study of influence of language upon thought and of the science of symbolism*, 296–336. New York: Harcourt, Brace & Co.

Marsden, Sharon & Janet Holmes. 2014. Talking to the elderly in New Zealand residential care settings. *Journal of Pragmatics* 64. 17–34.

Marson, Stephen M. & Rasby M. Powell. 2014. Goffman and the infantilization of elderly persons: A theory in development. *Journal of Sociology & Social Welfare* 41(4). 143–158.

Marvel, M. Kim, Ronald M. Epstein, Kristine Flowers & Howard B. Beckman. 1999. Soliciting the patient's agenda: Have we improved? *JAMA* 281(3). 283–287.

Masuda, Hiroya (ed.). 2015. *Tōkyō shōmetsu: kaigo hatan to chihō ijū* [Extinction of Tokyo: Care collapse and regional migration]. Tokyo: Chūō kōron.

Matsukawa, Miki & Yuki Morimoto. 2016. Iryō/kaigo no gaikokujin muzukashii teichaku [Nursing and care foreigners' difficulties to settle down]. *Asahi Shimbun*, 18 September.

Matsumoto, Yoshiko. 1985. A sort of speech act qualification in Japanese: *Chotto*. *Journal of Asian Culture* 9. 143–159.

Matsumoto, Yoshiko. 1988. Reexamination of the universality of face: Politeness phenomena in Japanese. *Journal of Pragmatics* 12(4). 403–426.

Matsumoto, Yoshiko. 2001. *Tyotto*: Speech act qualification in Japanese revisited. *Japanese Language and Literature* 35(1). 1–16.

Matsumoto, Yoshiko. 2011. Reframing to regain identity with humor: What conversations with friends suggest for communication in elderly care. In P. Backhaus (ed.), *Communication in elderly care: Cross-cultural perspectives*. 145–165. London & New York: Continuum.

Matsumoto, Yoshiko. 2014. Context in constructions: Variation in Japanese non-subject honorifics. In K. Kabata & T. Ono (eds.), *Usage-based approaches to Japanese grammar: Toward the understanding of human languages*, 261–278. Amsterdam & Philadelphia: Benjamins.

Matsunaga, Mikie & Satomi Iseki. 2004. Ninchishō kōreisha no komyunikēshon ryō to kanjō no bunseki [Analysis of communication quantity and feelings of older people with dementia]. *Niimi kōritsu tanki daigaku kiyō* 25. 171–177. http://ci.nii.ac.jp/naid/110004614096 (accessed 31 August 2016).

Matsuyama, Ikuo. 2006. Ninchishō kōreisha to no komyunikēshon ni tai suru kaigo shokuin no ninshiki [Care workers' awareness of communication with dementia patients]. *Saga daigaku bunka kyōiku gakubu kenkyū ronbunshū* 10(2). 181–188. http://ci.nii.ac.jp/naid/110004304594 (accessed 31 August 2016).

Maynard, Senko K. 1991. Pragmatics of discourse modality: A case of *da* and *desu/masu* forms in Japanese. *Journal of Pragmatics* 15(6). 551–582.

Maynard, Senko K. 2001. Falling in love with style: Expressive functions of stylistic shifts in a Japanese television drama series. *Functions of Language* 8(1). 1–39.

Maynard, Senko K. 2004. Poetics of style mixture: Emotivity, identity, and creativity in Japanese writings. *Poetics* 32(5). 387–409.

McCarthy, Michael. 2000. Mutual captive audiences: Small talk and the genre of close-contact service encounters. In J. Coupland (ed.), *Small talk*, 85–109. Essex: Pearson Education.

McCarthy, Michael & Anne O'Keeffe. 2003. What's in a name? Vocatives in casual conversation and radio phone-in calls. In P. Leistyna & C.F. Meyer (eds.), *Corpus analysis: Language structure and language use*, 153–185. Amsterdam & New York: Rodopi.

McClure, William. 2000. *Using Japanese: A guide to contemporary usage.* Cambridge & New York: Cambridge University Press.

McDowell, Joanne. 2015a. Masculinity and non-traditional occupations: Men's talk in women's work. *Gender, Work and Organization* 22(3). 273–291.

McDowell, Joanne. 2015b. Talk in feminised occupations: Exploring male nurses' linguistic behaviour. *Gender and Language* 9(3). 365–389.

McGloin, Naomi H. 1998. *Hai* and *ee*: An interactional analysis. In N. Akatsuka, H. Hoji, S. Iwasaki, S. Sohn & S. Strauss (eds.), *Japanese/Korean Linguistics* (Vol.7), 105–120. Stanford: Center for the Study of Language and Information.

McGloin, Naomi H. 2002. Markers of epistemic vs. affective stances: *Desyoo* vs. *zyanai*. In N.M. Akatsuka & S. Strauss (eds.), *Japanese/Korean Linguistics* (Vol.10), 136–149. Stanford: Center for the Study of Language and Information.

McLean, Athena. 2007. *The person in dementia: A study of nursing home care in the U.S.* Toronto: Broadview Press.

Megumi, Maeri. 2002. The switching between *desu/masu* form and plain form: From the perspective of turn construction. In N.M. Akatsuka & S. Strauss (eds.), *Japanese/Korean Linguistics* (Vol.10), 206–219. Stanford: Center for the Study of Language and Information.

Meißner, Anne. 2005. Das Problem der Anredeformen in der Pflege: Du oder Sie? In A. Abt-Zegelin & M.W. Schnell (eds.), *Sprache und Pflege* (Second edition), 45–49. Bern: Huber.

Menz, Florian & Ali Al-Roubaie. 2008. Interruptions, status and gender in medical interviews: The harder you brake, the longer it takes. *Discourse & Society* 19(5). 645–666.

Menz, Florian & Luzia Plansky. 2014. Time pressure and digressive speech patterns in doctor–patient consultations: Who is to blame? In E.-M. Graf, M. Sator & T. Spranz-Fogasy (eds.), *Discourses of helping professions*, 257–287. Amsterdam & Philadelphia: Benjamins.

MHLW (Ministry of Health, Labour and Welfare). 2016a. Heisei 26 nendo kaigo hoken jigyō jōkyō hōkoku (nenpō) no pointo [Main points of the 2014 report on the situation of care insurance projects]. http://www.mhlw.go.jp/topics/kaigo/osirase/jigyo/14/dl/h26_point.pdf (accessed 31 August 2016).

MHLW (Ministry of Health, Labour and Welfare). 2016b. Heisei 26 nendo kaigo hoken jigyō jōkyō hōkoku (nenpō): Hōkokusho no gaiyō [2014 report on the situation of care insurance projects: Overview]. http://www.mhlw.go.jp/topics/kaigo/osirase/jigyo/14/dl/h26_gaiyou.pdf (accessed 31 August 2016).

Miyake, Kazuko. 2001. 'Hai', 'ee', 'un' no gengo kōdō [The linguistic behaviour of 'hai', 'ee', and 'un']. *Dai 13 kai Nihongo kyōiku renraku kaigi hōkoku/happyō ronbunshū*. 49–56.

Miyake, Kazuko. 2009. Shazai mēru o meguru taijin kankei chōsei kōdō [The adjustment of interpersonal relationships in apology mails]. *Media to kotoba* 4. 158–188.

Mizutani, Osamu & Nobuko Mizutani. 1987. *How to be polite in Japanese*. Tokyo: Japan Times.

Mondada, Lorenza. 2014. Requesting immediate action in the surgical operation room: Time, embodied resources and praxeological embeddedness. In P. Drew & E. Couper-Kuhlen (eds.), *Requesting in social interaction*, 269–302. Amsterdam & Philadelphia: Benjamins.

Morikawa, Mie. 2014. Towards community-based integrated care: Trends and issues in Japan's long-term care policy. *International Journal of Integrated Care* 14. http://www.ijic.org/articles/10.5334/ijic.1066/ (accessed 31 August 2016).

Morita, Emi. 2005. *Negotiation of contingent talk: The Japanese interactional particles ne and sa*. Amsterdam & Philadelphia: Benjamins.

Muguruma, Yumi. 2012. *Odoroki no kaigo minzokugaku* [Care ethnography of surprises]. Tokyo: Igaku shoin.

Murata, Kazuyo. 2004. Terebi komāsharu no kōkando: sedaibetsu gengo sutoratejī no shiten kara [Favourability of TV commercials: From the viewpoint of generation specific strategies]. *Media to kotoba* 1. 2–35.

Murata, Kumiko. 1994. Intrusive or co-operative? A cross-cultural study of interruption. *Journal of Pragmatics* 21(4). 385–400.

Murray, Thomas E. 2002. A new look at address in American English: The rules have changed. *Names* 50(1). 43–61.

Nagakura, Katsue. 2016. Robotto ga kaigo suru hi ga yatte kuru [The day is coming when robots will do care]. *Shūkan Asahi*, 25 March, p.50.

Nagatomi, Satoko. 2012. Shin-keigo 'ssu' ni mirareru danjosa [Gender differences in the new honorific *ssu*]. *Shakai shisutemu kenkyū* 25. 129–147.

Naitō, Katsuo. 2006. Ninchishō kaigo ni okeru komyunikēshon ni kan suru kenkyū [Research on communication in dementia care]. (*Nihon daigaku bunri gakubu jinbun gakka kenkyūjo*) *Kenkyū kiyō* 72. 101–112.

Nakamura, Keiko. 2001. The acquisition of polite language by Japanese children. In K.E. Nelson & A. Aksu-Koç (eds.), *Children's language* (Vol.10), 93–112. Mahwah: Erlbaum.

Nakamura, Momoko. 2007. *'Sei' to Nihongo* [Gender and Japanese]. Tokyo: NHK Books.

Nakamura, Momoko. 2009. Language as heterosexual resource. *Shizen, ningen, shakai* 47. 1–23.

Nakayama, Akiko. 2003. *Shitashisa no komyunikēshon* [Communication of closeness]. Tokyo: Kuroshio.

Nguyen, Hanh Thi & Minh Thi Thuy Nguyen. 2016. 'But please can I play with the iPad?' The development of request negotiation practices by a four-year-old child. *Journal of Pragmatics* 101. 66–82.

Nishizaka, Aug. 2007. Kōi rensa no naka no keitai to jōtai [Formal and plain style in action chains]. *Meiji gakuin daigaku daigakuin shakaigaku kenkyūka shakaigaku senkō kiyō* 31. 55–78.

Nishizaka, Aug. 2014. Sustained orientation to one activity in multiactivity during prenatal ultrasound examinations. In P. Haddington, T. Keisanen, L. Mondada & M. Nevile (eds.), *Multiactivity in social interaction: Beyond multitasking*, 79–107. Amsterdam & Philadelphia: Benjamins.

Niyekawa, Agnes M. 1991. *Minimum essential politeness: A guide to the Japanese honorific language*. Tokyo: Kodansha.

Nofsinger, Robert E. 1991. *Everyday conversation*. Newbury Park, London, Los Angeles: Sage.

Noguchi, Mary Goebel. 2001. Introduction: The crumbling of a myth. In M. Goebel Noguchi & S. Fotos (eds.), *Studies in Japanese bilingualism*, 1–23. Clevedon: Multilingual Matters.

Norrby, Catrin & Camilla Wide. 2015. *Address practice as social action: European perspectives*. Houndmills: Palgrave Macmillan.

Norrby, Catrin, Camilla Wide, Jenny Nilsson & Jan Lindström. 2015. Address and interpersonal relationships in Finland–Swedish and Sweden–Swedish service encounters. In C. Norrby & C. Wide (eds.), *Address practice as social action: European perspectives*, 75–96. Houndmills: Palgrave Macmillan.

Nussbaum, Jon F. 1991. Communication, language and the institutionalized elderly. *Ageing & Society* 11(2). 149–165.

Nussbaum, Jon F. 1993. The communicative impact of institutionalization for the elderly: The admission process. *Journal of Aging Studies* 7(3). 237–246.

Obana, Yasuko. 2016. Speech level shifts in Japanese: A different perspective. *Pragmatics* 26(2). 247–290.

O'Connor, Brian P. & Holly Rigby. 1996. Perceptions of baby talk, frequency of receiving baby talk, and self-esteem among community and nursing home residents. *Psychology and Aging* 11(1). 147–154.

Ohwa, Mie & Li-Mei Chen. 2012. Balancing long-term care in Japan. *Journal of Gerontological Social Work* 55(7). 659–672.

Okamoto, Noriko. 1997. Kyōshitsu danwa ni okeru buntai shifuto no shihyōteki kinō: teineitai to futsūtai no tsukaiwake [Indexical functions of speech level shift in classroom discourse: Differentiating between formal and plain style]. *Nihongogaku* 6(3). 39–51.

Okamoto, Shigeko. 1995. 'Tasteless' Japanese: Less 'feminine' speech among young Japanese women. In K. Hall & M. Bucholtz (eds.), *Gender articulated: Language and the socially constructed self*, 297–325. New York: Routledge.

Okamoto, Shigeko. 1998. The use and non-use of honorifics in sales talk in Kyoto and Osaka: Are they rude or friendly? In N. Akatsuka, H. Hoji, S. Iwasaki, S.-O. Sohn & S. Strauss (eds.), *Japanese/Korean Linguistics* (Vol.7), 141–157. Stanford: Center for the Study of Language and Information.

Okamoto, Shigeko. 1999. Situated politeness: Coordinating honorific and non-honorific expressions in Japanese conversations. *Pragmatics* 9(1). 51–74.

Okamoto, Shigeko. 2016. Variability and multiplicity in the meanings of stereotypical gendered speech in Japanese. *East Asian Pragmatics* 1(1). 5–37.

Onoda, Takao. 2007. Kōreisha to herupā no kaiwa no tokuchō ni tsuite [On the characteristics of talk between elderly person and home helper]. *Tokoha gakuen tanki daigaku kenkyū kiyō* 38. 21–40. http://ci.nii.ac.jp/naid/110009435870 (accessed 31 August 2016).

Onoda, Takao. 2008. Kōreisha to herupā/kea mane to no kaiwa ni tsuite [On talk between elderly person and home helper/care manager]. *Tokoha gakuen tanki daigaku kenkyū kiyō* 39. 25–39. http://ci.nii.ac.jp/naid/110007659704 (accessed 31 August 2016).

Onoda, Takao. 2009. Kōreisha to kea mane to no kaiwa: rihabiri ni teikō suru yōshien kōreisha no kēsu ni tsuite [Talk between elderly person and care manager: When the person in need of care shows resistance against rehabilitation]. *Tokoha gakuen tanki daigaku kenkyū kiyō* 40. 29–39. http://ci.nii.ac.jp/naid/110007667378 (accessed 31 August 2016).

Onoda, Takao. 2010. 'Kōreisha–herupā' to 'kōreisha–keamane' no kotoba no hikaku: kaiwa no naka de no 'shikō yōshiki' to 'keiken' ni tsuite [Comparing the speech of elderly person–helper and elderly person–care manager: Mindsets and experiences inside conversation]. *Tokoha gakuen tanki daigaku kenkyū kiyō* 41. 37–44. http://ci.nii.ac.jp/naid/110008146879 (accessed 31 August 2016).

Onoda, Takao. 2011. Hatsuwa-ryō no suii kara mita ninchishō kōreisha to herupā to no kaiwa [Talk between elderly person with dementia and helper as seen from the change in number of utterances]. *Tokoha gakuen tanki daigaku kenkyū kiyō* 42. 1–14. http://ci.nii.ac.jp/naid/110008919216 (accessed 31 August 2016).

Onoda, Takao. 2013. Kōreisha no hanashi o monogatariteki na hyōgen yōshiki toshite rikai suru koto [Understanding an elderly person's speech as a narrative form of expression]. *Tokoha gakuen tanki daigaku kenkyū kiyō* 44. 1–18. http://ci.nii.ac.jp/naid/110009794984 (accessed 31 August 2016).

Onoda, Takao. 2014. Kaigo to komyunikēshon: hōmu herupā to no kaiwa [Care communication: Talk with the home helper]. *Nihongogaku* 33(11). 20–30.

Onoda, Takao. 2016a. Kaigo to kotoba dai 1 kai: kaigo ni totte no kotoba no kadai [Care and language 1: Topics in language for care]. *Nihongogaku* 35(6). 82–87.

Onoda, Takao. 2016b. Kaigo to kotoba dai 2 kai: kōreisha kaigo no kotoba no yōshiki [Care and language 2: The style of eldercare language]. *Nihongogaku* 35(9). 82–87.

Onoda, Takao. 2016c. Kaigo to kotoba dai 3 kai: hōmu herupā to kaiwa [Care and language 3: Conversations with home helpers]. *Nihongogaku* 35(9). 70–75.

Onoda, Takao. 2016d. Kaigo to kotoba saishūkai [Care and language, final installment]. *Nihongogaku* 35(12). 164–169.

Orpett Long, Susan. 2008. Social change and caregiving of the elderly. In F. Coulmas, H. Conrad, A. Schad-Seifert & G. Vogt (eds.), *The demographic challenge: A handbook about Japan*, 201–215. Leiden & Boston: Brill.

Orpett Long, Susan & Phyllis B. Harris. 1997. Caring for bedridden elderly: Ideals, realities, and social change in Japan. In S. Formanek & S. Linhart (eds.), *Aging: Asian concepts and experiences past and present*, 347–367. Vienna: Verlag der Österreichischen Wissenschaften.

Oshima, Sae & Jürgen Streeck. 2015. Coordinating talk and practical action: The case of hair salon service assessments. *Pragmatics and Society* 6(4). 538–564.

Ōta, Hitoshi & Haruki Miyoshi (eds.). 2005. *Jitsuyō kaigo jiten* [Practical care encyclopaedia]. Tokyo: Kodansha.

Ōtani, Shinya. 2004. Gaikokujin kaigo rōdōsha ukeire no mae ni: kōreisha kaigo genba ni okeru komyunikēshon [In advance of taking in foreign care workers: Communication in the care setting]. *Tabunka shakai to ryūgakusei kōryū* 8. 85–95.

Owada, Takeshi & Maki Kagaya. 2008. Hōmu herupā ni okeru seikatsu enjo toshite no komyunikēshon sukiru: Aomori-ken nai ni okeru hōmu herupā no ankēto chōsa kekka o tōshite [Home helpers' communication skills as living support: Results of a questionnaire survey of home helpers in Aomori Prefecture]. *Aomori kenritsu hoken daigaku zasshi* 9(1). 21–28. http://ci.nii.ac.jp/naid/110006978316 (accessed 31 August 2016).

Ozawa, Martha N. & Shingo Nakayama. 2005. Long-term care insurance in Japan. *Journal of Aging & Social Policy* 17(3). 61–84.

Peng, Ito. 2008. Ageing and the social security system. In F. Coulmas, H. Conrad, A. Schad-Seifert & G. Vogt (eds.), *The demographic challenge: A handbook about Japan*, 1033–1047. Leiden & Boston: Brill.

Persson, Tove & David Wästerfors. 2009. 'Such trivial matters': How staff account for restrictions of residents' influence in nursing homes. *Journal of Aging Studies* 23(1). 1–11.

Pizziconi, Barbara. 2003. Re-examining politeness, face and the Japanese language. *Journal of Pragmatics* 35(10/11). 1471–1506.

Pizziconi, Barbara. 2011. Honorifics: The cultural specificity of a universal mechanism in Japanese. In D.Z. Kádár & S. Mills (eds.), *Politeness in East Asia*, 45–70. Cambridge & New York: Cambridge University Press.

Placencia, María Elena. 2004. Rapport-building activities in corner shop interactions. *Journal of Sociolinguistics* 8(2). 215–245.

Placencia, María Elena. 2015. Address forms and relational work in e-commerce: The case of service encounter interactions in MercadoLibre Ecuador. In M. de la O Hernández-López & L. Fernández-Amaya (eds.), *A multidisciplinary approach to service encounters*, 37–64. Leiden & Boston: Brill.

Pomerantz, Anita. 1984a. Agreeing and disagreeing with assessments: Some features of preferred/dispreferred turn shapes. In J.M. Atkinson & J. Heritage (eds.), *Structures of social action*, 57–101. Cambridge: Cambridge University Press.

Pomerantz, Anita. 1984b. Pursuing a response. In J.M. Atkinson & J. Heritage (eds.), *Structures of social action*, 152–164. Cambridge: Cambridge University Press.

Posenau, André. 2013. Schwierige Momente während der Morgenpflege mit angepasster Kommunikation besser bewältigen. *Pflegezeitschrift: Fachzeitschrift für stationäre und ambulante Pflege* 66(2). 76–79.

Posenau, André. 2014. *Analyse der Kommunikation zwischen dementen Bewohnern und dem Pflegepersonal während der Morgenpflege im Altenheim.* Mannheim: Verlag für Gesprächsforschung. http://www.verlag-gespraechsforschung.de/2014/posenau.html (accessed 31 August 2016).

Pufahl Bax, Ingrid. 1986. How to assign work in an office: A comparison of spoken and written directives in American English. *Journal of Pragmatics* 10(6). 673–692.

Ragan, Sandra L. 1990. Verbal play and multiple goals in the gynaecological exam interaction. In N. Coupland & T. Revenson (eds.), *Multiple goals in discourse*, 67–84. Clevedon: Multilingual Matters.

Ragan, Sandra L. 2000. Sociable talk in women's healthcare contexts. In J. Coupland (ed.), *Small talk*, 269–287. Essex: Pearson Education.

Rauniomaa, Mirka & Tiina Keisanen. 2012. Two multimodal formats for responding to requests. *Journal of Pragmatics* 44(6/7). 829–842.

Rendle-Short, Johanna. 2007. 'Catherine, you're wasting your time': Address terms within the Australian political interview. *Journal of Pragmatics* 39(9). 1503–1525.

Riesco Bernier, Silvia. 2008. The discourse–grammar interface of regulatory teacher talk in the EFL classroom. In J. Romero-Trillo (ed.), *Pragmatics and corpus linguistics: A mutualistic entente*, 235–262. Berlin & New York: De Gruyter.

Robinson, Jeffrey D. 1998. Getting down to business: Talk, gaze, and body orientation during openings in doctor–patient consultations. *Human Communication Research* 25(1). 97–123.

Robinson, Jeffrey D. 2001. Closing medical encounters: Two physician practices and their implications for the expression of patients' unstated concerns. *Social Science & Medicine* 53(5). 639–656.

Robinson, Jeffrey D. 2013. Overall structural organization. In J. Sidnell & T. Stivers (eds.), *The handbook of conversation analysis*, 257–280. Malden, Oxford, West Sussex: Blackwell.

Ruhleder, Karen & Brigitte Jordan. 2001. Co-constructing non-mutual realities: Delay-generated trouble in distributed interaction. *Computer Supported Cooperative Work* 10(1). 113–138.

Ryan, Ellen B., Kerry Byrne, Hendrika Spykerman & J.B. Orange. 2005. Evidencing Kitwood's personhood strategies: Conversation as care in dementia. In B. Davis (ed.), *Alzheimer talk, text and context: Enhancing communication*, 18–36. New York: Palgrave Macmillan.

Ryan, Ellen B., Janet M. Hamilton & Sheree Kwong See. 1994. Patronizing the old: How do younger and older adults respond to baby talk in the nursing home? *International Journal of Aging and Human Development* 39(1). 21–32.

Ryan, Ellen B., Mary L. Hummert & Linda H. Boich. 1995. Communication predicaments of aging: Patronizing behavior toward older adults. *Journal of Language and Social Psychology* 14(1/2). 144–166.

Ryvicker, Miriam. 2009. Preservation of self in the nursing home: Contradictory practices within two models of care. *Journal of Aging Studies* 23(1). 12–23.

Sachweh, Svenja. 1998. Granny darling's nappies: Secondary babytalk in German nursing homes for the aged. *Journal of Applied Communication Research* 26(1). 52–65.

Sachweh, Svenja. 2000. *'Schätzle hinsitze!' Kommunikation in der Altenpflege*. Frankfurt: Lang.

Sachweh, Svenja. 2003. 'So frau Adams, guck mal, ein feines bac-spray, gut': Charakteristische Merkmale der Kommunikation zwischen Pflegepersonal und Bewohnerinnen in einem Altenpflegeheim. In R. Fiehler & C. Thimm (eds.), *Sprache und Kommunikation im Alter*, 143–160. Radolfzell: Verlag für Gesprächsforschung. http://www.verlag-gespraechsforschung.de/2004/alter/143–160.pdf (accessed 31 August 2016).

Sachweh, Svenja. 2005. *'Noch ein Löffelchen?' Effektive Kommunikation in der Altenpflege* (Second edition). Bern: Huber.

Sacks, Harvey, Emanuel A. Schegloff & Gail Jefferson. 1974. A simplest systematics for the organization of turn-taking in conversation. *Language* 50(4). 696–735.

Saito, Junko. 2010. Subordinates' use of Japanese plain forms: An examination of superior–subordinate interactions in the workplace. *Journal of Pragmatics* 42(12). 3271–3282.

Saito, Junko. 2011. Managing confrontational situations: Japanese male superiors' interactional styles in directive discourse in the workplace. *Journal of Pragmatics* 43(6). 1689–1706.

Salari, Sonia M. 2005. Infantilization as elder mistreatment: Evidence from five adult day care centers. *Journal of Elder Abuse & Neglect* 17(4). 53–91.

Salari, Sonia M. & Melinda Rich. 2001. Social and environmental infantilization of aged persons: Observations in two adult day care centers. *International Journal of Aging & Human Development* 52(2). 115–135.

Sasa, Sumiko. 2002. 'Desu/masu' hyōgen no tsukawarekata [Usage of *desu/masu* expressions]. In Gendai Nihongo kenkyūkai (ed.), *Dansei no kotoba: Shokuba-hen* [Men's language: Workplace edition], 75–87. Tokyo: Hituzi.

Sassen, Claudia. 2005. *Linguistic dimensions of crisis talk: Formalising structures in a controlled language.* Amsterdam & Philadelphia: Benjamins.

Schegloff, Emanuel A. 1968. Sequencing in conversational openings. *American Anthropologist* 70(6). 1075–1095.

Schegloff, Emanuel A. 1987. Recycled turn beginnings. In G. Button & J. Lee (eds.), *Talk and social organization,* 70–85. Clevedon: Multilingual Matters.

Schegloff, Emanuel A. 2000. Overlapping talk and the organization of turn-taking for conversation. *Language in Society* 29(1). 1–63.

Schegloff, Emanuel A. 2002. Accounts of conduct in interaction: Interruption, overlap and turn-taking. In J.H. Turner (ed.), *Handbook of sociological theory,* 287–321. New York: Plenum.

Schegloff, Emanuel A. 2004. On dispensability. *Research on Language and Social Interaction* 37(2). 95–149.

Schegloff, Emanuel A. 2007. *Sequence organization in interaction: A primer in conversation analysis* (Vol.1). Cambridge & New York: Cambridge University Press.

Schegloff, Emanuel A. & Harvey Sacks. 1973. Opening up closings. *Semiotica* 8(4). 289–327.

Sealey, Alison. 1999. 'Don't be cheeky': Requests, directives and being a child. *Journal of Sociolinguistics* 3(1). 24–40.

Shibatani, Masayoshi. 2001. Honorifics. In R. Mesthrie (ed.), *Concise encyclopedia of sociolinguistics,* 552–559. Oxford: Elsevier.

Shibuya, Hiroko, Chikara Miyoshi & Sachio Kumaki. 2008. Komyunikēshon no mondai ni tai suru kaigo shokuin no taisho purosesu no kentō: guraundeddo seorī ni yoru tokubetsu yōgo rōjin hōmu no shokuin/riyōsha kankei no bunseki [Studying care workers' coping process with communication problems: A grounded theory analysis of relationships between care workers and users in a nursing home]. *Rikkyō daigaku rinshō shinrigaku kenkyū* 2. 39–53.

Shimada, Shingo & Christian Tagsold. 2006. *Alternde Gesellschaften im Vergleich: Solidarität und Pflege in Deutschland und Japan.* Bielefeld: Transcript.

Shimanouchi, Setsu. 1986. Pākinson-byō kanja no shakai kankyō jōken to zaitaku kea kadai/yōken ni kan suru kenkyū [Study on the social environment and issues of in-home care for Parkinson patients]. *Shōwa igakukai zasshi* 46(2). 189–201. http://ci.nii.ac.jp/naid/130001826999 (accessed 31 August 2016).

Shioda, Takehiro. 2016. 'Sasete idatakimasu' ni tsuite kakasete itadakimasu [Taking the liberty to write on 'taking the liberty to']. In NHK Hōsō bunka kenkyūjo (ed.), *Hōsō kenkyū to chōsa* [NHK monthly report on broadcast research], 66(9). 26–41.

Simpson, Ruth. 2004. Masculinity at work: The experiences of men in female dominated occupations. *Work, Employment and Society* 18(2). 349–368.

Skovdahl, Kirsti, Annica Larsson Kihlgren & Mona Kihlgren. 2003. Dementia and aggressiveness: Video recorded morning care from different care units. *Journal of Clinical Nursing* 12(6). 888–898.

Slobin, Dan I., Stephen H. Miller & Lyman W. Porter. 1968. Forms of address and social relations in a business organization. *Journal of Personality and Social Psychology* 8(3). 289–293.

Smith, Janet S. 1992. Women in charge: Politeness and directives in the speech of Japanese women. *Language in Society* 21(1). 59–82.

Smith, Pam. 1992. *The emotional labour of nursing: Its impact on interpersonal relations, management and the educational environment in nursing.* London: Macmillan.

Smith, Pam. 2012. *The emotional labour of nursing revisited: Can nurses still care?* London: Palgrave Macmillan.

Smithers, Janice. 1977. Dimensions of senility. *Urban Life* 6(3). 251–276.

Sodei, Takako. 1995. Care of the elderly: A women's issue. In K. Fujimura-Fanselow & A. Kameda (eds.), *Japanese women: New feminist perspectives on the past, present, and future*, 213–228. New York: The Feminist Press.

Somera, Rene D. 1995. *Bordered aging: Ethnography of daily life in a Filipino home for the aged.* Manila: De La Salle University Press.

Somera, Rene D. 1997. Language, context, and elderly rights: Linguistic ageism in a Filipino home for the aged. *BOLD: Quarterly Journal of the International Institute on Ageing* 8. 16–25.

Sorjonen, Marja-Leena & Liisa Raevaara. 2014. On the grammatical form of requests at the convenience store: Requesting as embodied action. In P. Drew & E. Couper-Kuhlen (eds.), *Requesting in social interaction*, 243–268. Amsterdam & Philadelphia: Benjamins.

Staples, Shelley. 2015. *The discourse of nurse–patient interactions: Contrasting the communicative styles of U.S. and international nurses.* Amsterdam & Philadelphia: Benjamins.

Stevanovic, Melisa & Chiara Monzoni. 2016. On the hierarchy of interactional resources: Embodied and verbal behavior in the management of joint activities with material objects. *Journal of Pragmatics* 103. 15–32.

Stivers, Tanya. 2004. 'No no no' and other types of multiple sayings in social interaction. *Human Communication Research* 30(2). 260–293.

Stivers, Tanya. 2013. Sequence organization. In J. Sidnell & T. Stivers (eds.), *The handbook of conversation analysis*, 191–209. Malden, Oxford, West Sussex: Blackwell.

Stivers, Tanya & Federico Rossano. 2010. Mobilizing response. *Research on Language and Social Interaction* 43(1). 3–31.

Street, Richard L. &. David B. Buller. 1988. Patients' characteristics affecting physician–patient nonverbal communication. *Human Communication Research* 15(1). 60–90.

SturtzSreetharan, Cindi L. 2006. Gentlemanly gender? Japanese men's use of clause-final politeness in casual conversations. *Journal of Sociolinguistics* 10(1). 70–92.

SturtzSreetharan, Cindi L. 2009. '*Ore*' and '*omae*': Japanese men's use of first- and second-person pronouns. *Pragmatics* 19(2). 253–278.

Sudo, Jun. 2005. Kaiwa sankasha no shakaiteki kankei ni yoru kandōshi no onseiteki tokuchō: ōtō ni okeru 'a' no bariēshon [Phonetic characteristics of interjections as based on the speech participants' social relationship: Variation of *a* in responses]. *Shakai gengo kagaku* 8(1). 181–193. http://ci.nii.ac.jp/naid/110009570090 (accessed 31 August 2016).

Sugita, Yuko. 2004. *Gesprächserwartungen: Eine kontrastive Studie über die Gesprächsführung in deutschen und japanischen Telefonaten.* Frankfurt: Lang.

Sugita, Yuko. 2012. Minimal affect uptake in a pre-climax position of conversational 'scary' stories. *Journal of Pragmatics* 44(10). 1273–1289.

Sugiyama, Tomoko, Noriko Matsui, Hiroki Fukahori & Yuichi Sugai. 2008. Arutsuhaimā-gata chūki ninchishō kanja e no ADL kea ni tai suru teikō-ji ni okeru kea sutaffu no kakawari no tokusei [Characteristics of staff involvement when dealing with intermediate Alzheimer dementia patients' resistance toward ADL care]. *Iryō kango kenkū* 4(1). 1–9. http://ci.nii.ac.jp/naid/110006966298 (accessed 31 August 2016).

Suwa, Shigeki. 1996. *Zoku kaigo senmonshoku no tame no koekake/ōtō handobukku: komatta toki no hitokoto* [Handbook for care professionals on address and reply: Phrases when in trouble]. Tokyo: Chūō hōki.

Suzuki, Kenji, Tadashi Sotoyama & Ken Miura. 2002. Chihōsei kōreisha gurūpu hōmu ni okeru nyūkyosha no seikatsu to sutaffu no kea no sōgo shintō: chihōsei kōreisha no kea kankyō no arikata ni kan suru kenkyū (2) [Interpenetration of resident life and staff care in a group home for elderly people with dementia: Research on the care environment (2)]. *Nihon kenchiku gakkai keikakukei ronbunshū* 552. 125–131. http://ci.nii.ac.jp/naid/110004658078 (accessed 31 August 2016).

Suzuki, Ryota, Masaya Arai, Yoshihisa Sato, Taichi Yamada, Yoshinori Kobayashi, Yoshinori Kuno, Satoshi Miyazawa, Mihoko Fukushima, Keiichi Yamazaki & Akiko Yamazaki. 2015. Fukusū dōhansha to no gurūpu komyunikēshon o kōsatsu shita fukusū robotto kurumaisu shisutemu [Robotic wheelchair system allowing group communication among wheelchair users and accompanying persons]. *Denshi jōhō tsūshin gakkai ronbunshū* J98-A(1). 51–62. http://ci.nii.ac.jp/naid/120005575549 (accessed 31 August 2016).

Suzuki, Seiko. 2001. Kaigo fukushishoku no komyunikēshon sukiru ni kan suru kentō: jiko hyōka kara [Study on communication skills of care workers through self-estimations]. *Kaigo fukushigaku* 8(1). 71–78.

SWET (Society of Writers, Editors and Translators). 1998. *Japan style sheet: The SWET guide for writers, editors, and translators.* Berkeley: Stone Bridge Press.

Świtek, Beata. 2014. Representing the alternative: Demographic change, migrant eldercare workers, and national imagination in Japan. *Contemporary Japan* 26(2). 263–280. http://www.tandfonline.com/doi/abs/10.1515/cj-2014–0013 (accessed 24 January 2017).

Tachikawa, Kazumi. 2009. Kaigo shisetsu de no shokuji bamen ni okeru komyunikēshon ni tsuite: Gaikokujin kaigo rōdōsha ni tai suru Nihongo kyōiku ni mukete [On communication in care facilities during meal times: Addressing Japanese language education for foreign care workers]. *Ryūtsū keizai daigaku shakai gakubu ronsō* 20(1). 1–14. http://ci.nii.ac.jp/naid/110010007740 (accessed 31 August 2016).

Tachikawa, Kazumi. 2010. Kaigo katsudō to komyunikēshon: sono jittai to kenkyū kekka [Care activities and communication: Their actual condition and research results]. *Ryūtsū keizai daigaku shakai gakubu ronsō* 21(1). 29–43. http://ci.nii.ac.jp/naid/110010007772 (accessed 31 August 2016).

Tachikawa, Kazumi. 2011. Gaikokujin kaigo fukushi ukeire genba no jissai: Nihongo to Nihon bunka no mondai o chūshin ni [The reality of taking in foreign care workers: Focussing on the problem of Japanese language and culture]. *Ryūtsū keizai daigaku shakai gakubu ronsō* 21(2). 45–61. http://ci.nii.ac.jp/naid/110010007778 (accessed 31 August 2016).

Tachikawa, Kazumi. 2012. Kōreisha kaigo shisetsu ni okeru danwa no tokusei: kaigosha no komyunikēshon sutoratejī o megutte [Characteristics of discourse in eldercare facilities: Centring on care workers' communication skills]. *Ryūtsū keizai daigaku shakai gakubu ronsō* 23(1). 81–96. http://ci.nii.ac.jp/naid/110010007806 (accessed 31 August 2016).

Tachikawa, Kazumi. 2013. Kōreisha kaigo shisetsu no danwa ni miru komyunikēshon patān: gaikokujin kaigoshi ni tai suru Nihongo kyōiku e no ōyō e mukete [Communication patterns in eldercare facility discourse: Addressing Japanese language instruction for foreign care workers]. *Ryūtsū keizai daigaku shakai gakubu ronsō* 24(1). 95–112. http://ci.nii.ac.jp/naid/110010007822 (accessed 31 August 2016).

Tachikawa, Kazumi. 2015. Ibunka komyunikēshon kara kangaeru gaikokujin ikusei no tame no Nihongo kyōiku: kaigo genba ni okeru irai hyōgen ni kan suru ichi kōsatsu [Thinking about Japanese language teaching for foreign caregivers from the viewpoint of intercultural communication: Considerations on request expressions in care settings]. *Ryūtsū keizai daigaku shakai gakubu ronsō* 25(2). 49–74. http://ci.nii.ac.jp/naid/110010007846 (accessed 31 August 2016).

Takada, Akira & Tomoko Endo. 2015. Object transfer in request–accept sequence in Japanese caregiver–child interaction. *Journal of Pragmatics* 82. 52–66.

Takagi, Tomoyo. 2008. Sōgo kōi o seijo suru tetsuzuki toshite no ukete no hannō: chiryōteki mensetsu bamen de mochiirareru 'hai' o megutte [Recipient response as a method for ordering interaction: The use of *hai* in a therapy session]. *Shakai gengo kagaku* 10(2). 55–69. http://ci.nii.ac.jp/naid/110009570140 (accessed 31 August 2016).

Takamoto, Kaori. 2011. Ibunka kango/kaigo to komyunikēshon: EPA ni motozuku gaikokujin kangoshi/kaigoshi kōhosha no ukeire o megutte [Intercultural care and communication: Taking in foreign care workers on the basis of the EPA]. *Reitaku gakusai jānaru* 19(1). 33–43. http://ci.nii.ac.jp/naid/110008464082 (accessed 31 August 2016).

Takemura, Shinji, Michio Hashimoto, Wataru Koyano & Hisao Osada. 1999. Kaigo sābisu ga kōreisha ni oyobosu kōka ni kan suru kenkyū: tokubetsu yōgo rōjin hōmu ni okeru 'koekake' no kekka no kenshō [The effects of 'koekake' on the physical and mental status of elderly people in an eldercare facility]. *Rōnen shakai gakkai* 21(1). 15–25.

Takenoya, Miyuki. 2003. *Terms of address in Japanese: An interlanguage pragmatics approach*. Sapporo: Hokkaido University Press.

Taleghani-Nikazm, Carmen. 2006. *Request sequences: The intersection of grammar, interaction and social context*. Amsterdam & Philadelphia: Benjamins.

Tanaka, Hiroko. 2000. The particle *ne* as a turn-management device in Japanese conversation. *Journal of Pragmatics* 32(8). 1135–1176.

Tanaka, Hiromasa. 2011. Politeness in a Japanese intra-organisational meeting: Honorifics and socio-dialectal code switching. *Journal of Asian Pacific Communication* 21(1). 60–76.

Tanaka, Hiroshi. 2014. Kaigo shisetsu riyōsha to shokuin no komyunikēshon chōsa hōkoku [Survey report on communication between users and staff of a care facility]. *Komyunikēshon bunka* 8. 56–68.

Tanaka, Lidia. 2004. *Gender, language and culture: A study of Japanese television interview discourse*. Amsterdam & Philadelphia: Benjamins.

Tanaka, Lidia. 2010. Is formality relevant? Japanese tokens *hai, ee* and *un*. *Pragmatics* 20(2). 191–211.

Taniguchi, Maya. 2004. Nihongo no kōen no danwa ni okeru supīchi reberu shifuto no keitai to kinō [Forms and functions of speech level shift in discourse of lectures in Japanese]. *Waseda daigaku Nihongo kyōiku kenkyū* 4. 117–129. http://ci.nii.ac.jp/naid/110004627875 (accessed 31 August 2016).

Tannen, Deborah. 1987. Repetition in conversation: Toward a poetics of talk. *Language* 63. 574–605.

Tannen, Deborah. 1992. Interactional sociolinguistics. In W. Bright (ed.), *Oxford international encyclopedia of linguistics* (Vol.4), 9–12. Oxford & New York: Oxford University Press.

Taylor, Jenna. 2016. I need a coffee: Pragmalinguistic variation of requests in Starbucks service encounters. *IULC Working Papers* 15(1). 33–61. https://www.indiana.edu/~iulcwp/wp/article/view/15-02 (accessed 31 August 2016).

ten Have, Paul. 1991. Talk and institution: A reconsideration of the 'asymmetry' of doctor–patient interaction. In D. Boden & D. Zimmerman (eds.), *Talk and social structure*, 138–163. Cambridge: Polity Press.

Thang, Leng Leng. 2011. Aging and social welfare in Japan. In V.L. Bestor, T.C. Bestor & A. Yamagata (eds.), *Routledge handbook of Japanese culture and society*, 172–185. Abingdon & New York: Routledge.

Thimm, Caja. 1997. Sprache und Pflege: Überlegungen aus der Sicht der linguistischen Frauenforschung. In A. Zegelin (ed.), *Sprache und Pflege*, 67–76. Berlin & Wiesbaden: Ullstein-Mosby.

Thomas, Lois Helene. 1992. A comparison of the work of qualified nurses and nursing auxiliaries in primary, team and functional nursing wards. Dissertation thesis, Newcastle University. http://hdl.handle.net/10443/285 (accessed 31 August 2016).

Thornton, Robert & Leah L. Light. 2006. Language comprehension and production in normal aging. In J.E. Birren & K.W. Schaire (eds.), *Handbook of the psychology of aging* (Sixth edition), 261–287. Amsterdam: Elsevier.

Toerien, Merran & Celia Kitzinger. 2007. Emotional labour in action: Navigating multiple involvements in the beauty salon. *Sociology* 41(4). 645–662.

Togashi, Junichi. 2002. 'Hai' to 'un' no kankei o megutte [About 'hai' and 'un']. In Toshiyuki Tadanobu (ed.), *'Hai' to 'un' no gengogaku* [The linguistics of hai and un], 127–157. Tokyo: Hituzi.

Tranter, Nicolas & Mika Kizu. 2012. Modern Japanese. In N. Tranter (ed.), *The languages of Japan and Korea*, 268–312. London & New York: Routledge.

Traphagan, John W. 2000. *Taming oblivion: Aging bodies and the fear of senility in Japan*. Albany: State University of New York.

Traugott, Elisabeth C. & Richard B. Dasher. 2002. *Regularity in semantic change*. Cambridge: Cambridge University Press.

Tsuda, Sanae. 2010. Interpersonal functions of the polite forms *desu/masu* in Japanese conversations. *Intercultural Communication Studies* 19(3). 81–89. http://www.uri.edu/iaics/content/2010v19n3/06SanaeTsuda.pdf (accessed 31 August 2016).

Twine, Nanette. 1991. *Language and the modern state: The reform of written Japanese*. London: Routledge.

Udo, Mariko. 2007. Kansei o shintai de arawasu kotoba: gengo to ongaku to miburi ga chōwa suru hanchū [Language to express sensitivity through the body: A category that harmonises language, music, and gestures]. *Kōbe gengogaku ronsō* 5. 217–234. http://ci.nii.ac.jp/naid/110006867350 (accessed 31 August 2016).

Ueda, Naoko, Emiko Hujisawa, Nobuo Aoki, Hiromichi Hosoma, Yuri Yoshimura & Masaki Yoshimura. 2007. 'Nomazu ni kanda?' 'Kamazu ni nonda!': gurūpu hōmu ni okeru sōgo kōi [Chewed without swallowing? Swallowed without chewing! Interaction in a group home]. *Seisen ronsō* 15. 303–324. http://ci.nii.ac.jp/naid/110006966702 (accessed 31 August 2016).

Uehara, Satoshi. 2011. The socio-cultural motivation of referent honorifics in Korean and Japanese. In K.-U. Panther & G. Radden (eds.), *Motivation in grammar and the lexicon*, 191–212. Amsterdam & Philadelphia: Benjamins.

Ueno, Chizuko. 2011. *Kea no shakaigaku* [The sociology of care]. Tokyo: Ohta shuppan.

Usami, Mayumi (ed.). 1997. *Kotoba wa shakai o kaerareru* [Language can change society]. Tokyo: Akashi shoten.

Usami, Mayumi. 1999. Kōreisha to no komyunikēshon [Communication with elderly people]. In Tōkyō-to rōjin sōgo kenkyūjo (ed.), *Otoshiyori no komyunikēshon o kangaeru* [Thinking about communication with elderly people], 58–91. Tokyo: Tōkyō-to rōjin iryō sentā.

Usami, Mayumi. 2002. *Discourse politeness in Japanese conversation: Some implications for a universal theory of politeness.* Tokyo: Hituzi.

Usami, Mayumi. 2015. Nihongo no 'sutairu' ni kakawaru kenkyū no gaikan to tenbō: Nihongo kaiwa ni okeru supīchi reberu shifuto ni kan suru kenkyū o chūshin ni [On styles in Japanese language: Focusing on speech level shift in Japanese conversation]. *Shakai gengo kagaku* 18(1). 7–22.

Usami, Mayumi & Orie Endō. 1997. Kōreisha to gengo (2): kōreisha ni tai suru kotoba [Old people and language (2): Speech addressing the elderly]. *Nihongo* 10. 66–71.

Vine, Bernadette. 2004. *Getting things done at work: The discourse of power in work-place interaction.* Amsterdam & Philadelphia: Benjamins.

Vinkhuyzen, Erik & Margaret S. Szymanski. 2005. Would you like to do it yourself? Service requests and their non-granting responses. In K. Richards & P. Seedhouse (eds.), *Applying conversation analysis*, 91–106. New York: Palgrave Macmillan.

Vismans, Roel. 2015. Negotiating address in a pluricentric language: Dutch/Flemish. In C. Norrby & C. Wide (eds.), *Address practice as social action: European perspectives*, 13–23. Houndmills: Palgrave Macmillan.

Vogt, Gabriele. 2009. An invisible policy shift: International health-care migration to Japan. APSA 2009 Toronto Meeting Paper. http://ssrn.com/abstract=1448988 (accessed 31 August 2016).

Wadensten, Barbro. 2005. The content of morning time conversations between nursing home staff and residents. *Journal of Clinical Nursing* 14 (Issue Supplement s2). 84–89.

Wagnild, Gail & Roger Manning. 1985. Convey respect during bathing procedures. *Journal of Gerontological Nursing* 11(12). 6–10.

Ward, Richard, Antony A. Vass, Neeru Aggarwal, Cydonie Garfield & Beau Cybyk. 2008. A different story: Exploring patterns of communication in residential dementia care. *Ageing & Society* 28(5). 629–651.

Warren, Jane. 2006. Address pronouns in French: Variation within and outside the workplace. *Australian Review of Applied Linguistics* 29(2). 16.1–17 https://benjamins.com/#catalog/journals/aral.29.2.01war/fulltext (accessed 31 August 2016).

Watanabe, Atsuko. 2008. Kaigo shisetsu ni okeru komyunikēshon jiko hyōka no kōsatsu: gakusei to shisetsu shokuin no hikaku [Self-evaluations of communication in a care facility: Comparing students and care workers] (*Nagoya ryūjō tanki daigaku*) *Kenkyū kiyō* 30. 179–193. http://ci.nii.ac.jp/naid/110007040582 (accessed 31 August 2016).

Weigel, M. Margaret & Ronald M. Weigel. 1985. Directive use in a migrant agricultural community: A test of Ervin-Tripp's hypotheses. *Language in Society* 14(1). 63–79.

Weinhold, Christine. 1997. *Kommunikation zwischen Patienten und Pflegepersonal.* Bern: Huber.

Wells, Thelma J. 1980. *Problems in geriatric nursing care: A study of nurses' problems in care of old people in hospitals.* New York: Livingstone.

West, Candace. 1984. *Routine complications: Trouble with talk between doctors and patients.* Bloomington: Indiana University Press.

West, Candace. 1990. Not just 'doctors' orders': Directive–response sequences in patients' visits to women and men physicians. *Discourse & Society* 1(1). 85–112.

West, Candace & Don H. Zimmerman. 1977. Women's place in everyday talk: Reflections on parent–child interactions. *Social Problems* 24(5). 521–529.

Wetzel, Patricia. 2010. Public signs as narratives in Japan. *Japanese Studies* 30(3). 325–342.

Wierzbicka, Anna. 1991. *Cross-cultural pragmatics: The semantics of human interaction.* Berlin & New York: Mouton de Gruyter.

Wilkinson, Louise Cherry & Steven Calculator. 1982. Effective speakers: Students' use of language to request and obtain information in action in the classroom. In L.C. Wilkinson (ed.), *Communicating in the classroom*, 85–99. New York: Academic Press.

Williams, Christine L. (ed.). 1993. *Doing women's work: Men in non-traditional occupations.* London: Sage.

Williams, Kristine & Carol A.B. Warren. 2009. Communication in assisted living. *Journal of Aging Studies* 23. 24–36.

Wilson, Nick. 2010. Bros, boys and guys: Address term function and communities of practice in a New Zealand rugby team. *New Zealand English Journal* 24. 34–54.

Wood, Barbara & Royce Gardner. 1980. How children get their way: Directives in communication. *Communication Education* 29(3). 264–272.

Wood, Linda A. & Ellen B. Ryan. 1991. Talk to elders: Social structure, attitudes and forms of address. *Ageing & Society* 11(2). 167–187.

Wootton, Anthony J. 1981. Two request forms of four year olds. *Journal of Pragmatics* 5(6). 511–523.

Wright, Heather Harris (ed.). 2016. *Cognition, language and aging.* Amsterdam & Philadelphia: Benjamins.

Wu, Yongmei. 2004. *The care of the elderly in Japan.* London & New York: RoutledgeCurzon.

Yamada, Kiyomi & Kimiaki Nishida. 2007. Kaigo sutaffu ga ninchishō kōreisha ni mochiiru komyunikēshon gihō no tokuchō to sono kanren yōin [Characteristics and correlated factors of nursing assistants' communication strategies for persons with dementia]. *Nihon kango kenkyū gakkai zasshi* 30(4). 85–91. http://ci.nii.ac.jp/naid/130005143400 (accessed 31 August 2016).

Yamaguchi, Masataka. 1999. A critical study of discursive practices of 'othering' in construction of national identities: The case of learners of Japanese as a foreign language. Dissertation thesis, University of Georgia. http://hdl.handle.net/10724/22033 (accessed 31 August 2016).

Yamaguchi, Toshiko. 2007. *Japanese language in use: An introduction.* London & New York: Continuum.

Yamamoto, Mari. 2016. Sōgo kōi ni okeru kikite hannō toshite no 'un/hai' no tsukaiwake: 'teineisa' to kotonaru kanten kara [*Un/hai* as hearer's reaction in interaction: Viewpoints other than formality]. *Kokuritsu kokugo kenkyūjo ronshū* 10. 297–313. http://ci.nii.ac.jp/naid/120005702337 (accessed 31 August 2016).

Yamazaki, Keiichi, Michie Kawashima, Yoshinori Kuno, Naonori Akiya, Matthew Burdelski, Akiko Yamazaki & Hideaki Kuzuoka. 2007. Prior-to-request and request behaviors within elderly day care: Implications for developing service robots for use in multiparty settings. In L. Bannon, I. Wagner, C. Gutwin, R. Harper & K. Schmidt (eds.), *ECSCW 2007: Proceedings of the tenth European conference on computer supported cooperative work*, 61–78. London: Springer.

Yasutome, Takako. 2009. Kaigo/kango genba ni okeru gaikokujin rōdōsha no komyunikēshon ni kan suru kadai: Betonamu-jin kangoshi yōsei shien jigyō to keizai renkei kyōtei (EPA) ni yoru ukeire no hikaku o chūshin ni [Issues regarding communication of foreign care workers in care and nursing settings: Comparison of the EPA program with support programs for the training of Vietnamese nurses]. *Ryūtsū keizai daigaku shakai gakubu ronsō* 44(3). 229–240. http://ci.nii.ac.jp/naid/110010008000 (accessed 31 August 2016).

Ylänne-McEwen, Virpi. 2004. Shifting alignment and negotiating sociality in travel agency discourse. *Discourse Studies* 6(4). 517–533.

Yokoi, Mitsuharu. 2009. Kaigo jisshū ni okeru komyunikēshon gijutsu no shūtoku ni kan suru kenkyū [Research on the acquisition of communication skills in care training]. *Ōsaka taiiku daigaku tanki daigakubu kenkyū kiyō* 10. 33–45. http://ci.nii.ac.jp/naid/110007149574 (accessed 31 August 2016).

Yong, Vanessa & Yasuhiko Saito. 2012. National long-term care insurance policy in Japan a decade after implementation: Some lessons for aging countries. *Ageing International* 37(3). 271–284.

Yoshida, Seiko. 2007. Ninchishō kōreisha e no hōmon kaigoin no kakawari kōdō ni tsuite no ichi shiryō: chakudatsu bamen de no taiō o chūshin ni [Data on relational behavior of home helpers towards elderly persons with dementia: Focus on resistance to change clothes]. *Kaigo fukushigaku* 14(2). 175–180.

Yoshikawa, Yuki, Shinji Kato, Tetsuya Abe & Tomoyuki Yabuki. 2005. Mogi kaiwa bamen no VTR o mochiita kaigo shokuin no hatsuwa sutairu no hyōka [Evaluations of care workers' utterance style using video data of mock conversations]. *Nihon ninchishō kea gakkaishi* 4. 51–61.

Yoshikawa, Yuki, Shinji Kato, Mitsue Goto, Ai Honma & Kanako Sugiyama. 2004. Chihōsei kōreisha to no shōshūdan komyunikēshon ni okeru kaigo shokuin no yakuwari [Care workers' role in small-group communication with elderly people with dementia]. *Kōreisha chihō kaigo kenkyū/kenshū Sendai sentā kenkyū nenpō* 5. 133–145.

Yoshikawa, Yuki & Kuniaki Sugai. 2005. Ninchishō kōreisha ni tai suru kaigo shokuin no hatsuwa chōsetsu: hatsuwa tāgetto oyobi hatsuwasha no sai kara kentō [Care workers' speech accommodation for elderly with dementia: Focus on differences in utterance target and speaker]. *Komyunikēshon shōgaigaku* 22(1). 1–11. http://ci.nii.ac.jp/naid/10015684680 (accessed 31 August 2016).

Yoshitomi, Chie. 2009. Fukushi genba de motomerareru komyunikēshon nōryoku ni tsuite no ichi kōsatsu [Observation about communication skills in welfare settings]. *Ryūkoku kiyō* 31(1). 147–165. http://ci.nii.ac.jp/naid/110008719485 (accessed 31 August 2016).

Yuki, Yasuhiro. 2008. *Kaigo genba kara no kenshō* [Inspections from the care setting]. Tokyo: Iwanami.

Zwicky, Arnold. 1974. 'Hey, Whatsyourname'. In M. La Galy, R.A. Fox & A. Bruck (eds.), *Papers from the tenth regional meeting, Chicago Linguistic Society*, 787–801. Chicago: Chicago Linguistic Society.

Appendix 1
Note on transcription

Each transcribed line normally consists of two parts. The upper line gives the original Japanese utterance in romanised transliteration based on the modified Hepburn system (see closing paragraph of the introduction), the lower one an English approximation of it. In order to keep the transcripts maximally readable, I decided against adding an interlinear gloss. Where necessary, meta-comments on lexico-grammatical specifics are added in double brackets at the end of the English translation. Double brackets are also used to gloss exclamations, sighs, heave-hoes, and other material that proved difficult to replicate in English. No second line is given for "undecipherable" sounds.

List of transcription symbols and abbreviations used

?	rising intonation
,	continuing intonation
[	beginning of overlap
=	latched to previous utterance/line
(0.3)	pause of 0.3 seconds
(1.5, comment)	pause of 1.5 seconds plus meta-comment or explanation
((comment))	meta-comment or explanation
(text)	best guess about not clearly audible text
###	incomprehensible text (number of #s indicates approximate number of syllables)
°text°	spoken softly or whispered
tex:t	lengthening (number of colons indicates degree of lengthening)
tEXt	emphasis or non-standard accentuation
te/	halting or abrupt cutoff
Res	resident's speech
CW	care worker's speech
FN	addressee's first name
LN	addressee's last name

Appendix 2
Detailed table of contents of main text

Index